Human Growth and its Disorders

HUMAN GROWTH AND ITS DISORDERS

W. A. MARSHALL
Institute of Child Health
University of London

1977

ACADEMIC PRESS
London · New York · San Francisco
A Subsidiary of Harcourt Brace Jovanovich, Publishers

U.K. Edition published and distributed by
ACADEMIC PRESS INC. (LONDON) LTD.
24/28 Oval Road
London NW1

United States Edition published and distributed by
ACADEMIC PRESS INC.
111 Fifth Avenue
New York, New York 10003

Library of Congress Catalog Card Number: 77–71833
ISBN: 0–12–473950–4

Text set in 11/12 pt Monotype Baskerville, by W. S. Cowell Ltd., Ipswich
Printed in Great Britain by
Whitstable Litho Ltd., Whitstable, Kent.

Foreword

The Department of Growth and Development at the Institute of Child Health was formally established in 1957 when R. H. Whitehouse and I were invited by Professor Sir Alan Moncrieff to bring together our Harpenden Growth Study, then seven years old, and a second study of normal children begun at the Institute by Dr Frank Falkner, now Director of the Fels Research Institute, Ohio. Alan Moncrieff was convinced that auxology, the study of growth and development, was the basic science of paediatrics and should form the cornerstone of any real edifice of child health.

At first the Department stumbled along on less than the proverbial shoestring until in 1962 the Nuffield Foundation made us a magnificent grant totalling nearly a quarter of a million pounds. This enabled a real department to be built up, embracing experimental, behavioural and clinical auxology. Dr W. A. Marshall was the first to join us, together with Dr N. Blurton Jones, the childhood ethologist.

In 1963 Dr Marshall and I established a Growth Disorder Clinic at the Hospital for Sick Children and began a long and arduous campaign to convert our colleagues to the correctness of Alan Moncrieff's view. We had powerful allies, for our growth study was only one of a closely linked series in Brussels, London, Paris, Stockholm, Zurich, Dakar and Louisville, coordinated and cared for by the late Dr Nathalie Masse of the International Children's Centre, Paris. The directors of the Swiss and Swedish studies (Professors Andrea Prader and Petter Karlberg) were distinguished paediatricians whose influence greatly facilitated the emergence of paediatric auxology in Europe; and in North America Dr Falkner and his colleagues valiantly strove to direct their colleagues' attention to a field that was not currently fashionable.

This book represents, I think, a culmination of that campaign to bring auxology into the paediatric market place. Any paediatrician or family doctor who has read it will be sensible, I am sure, of the benefit that this new perspective and knowledge will bring to the children and adolescents he cares for. I heartily recommend it to all medical students, family doctors and paediatricians in training who can read simple, clear and concise English; I believe it should be an essential element in their course; and I am proud indeed to claim, in a sense, a share of its grandparentage.

July 1977   J. M. TANNER

Preface

Abnormal growth is often a presenting symptom of systemic disease which is a potential cause of handicap or death. Also, many basically healthy children whose growth-regulating mechanisms are impaired can now be treated very successfully. For example, growth hormone deficiency, whose diagnosis was only a matter of academic interest a generation ago, is now amenable to treatment which enables patients to take an entirely normal place in society. Nowadays any clinician who fails to recognise a child's abnormal growth, and have it properly investigated, is doing his patient a disservice. A thorough understanding of the ways in which growth is studied; how it may be modified by natural influences (either normal or pathological) and by medical intervention, is therefore an indispensible part of the modern paediatricians equipment. Here I use the word paediatrician in its widest sense, to include any physician concerned directly with the care of children whether in hospital, in the family setting, or at the level of the community physician.

The study of growth is largely concerned with variation, that is with the differences between individuals. The clinician may wish to know if the stature of his ten-year-old patient is within the normal range of variation for a child of this age and whether the child is currently growing at an acceptable speed. He can only answer this question by studying charts of tables which tell him the limits of variation in both stature and growth rate amongst normal children. This information, of course, can only be obtained by studying large and carefully selected samples of normal children who are representative of the population.

The creation, in this way, of 'growth standards' is also of fundamental importance to those responsible for monitoring the health and well-being of children and advising on the effectiveness of measures to improve their nutrition or freedom from disease. The monitoring of growth from this point of view is particularly important in developing countries. Repeated studies at intervals of five or ten years will reveal improvements (or the opposite) in children's growth. These changes are an important index in the general well-being of the population.

If the growth rates of children belonging to different racial, social, economic or geographical groups are compared, we can make inferences about the importance of these variables in regulating growth.

Educationalists, psychologists and workers in related fields, are familiar with the difficulties experienced by some children who are unusually short or strikingly tall by comparison with others of the same age.

Sometimes, as we shall see, a child's "bigness" or "smallness" in relation to his peers is only temporary because he is either more or less advanced in his progress towards his adult height than they are. Similarly, the development of the secondary sex character may be early or late. Obviously clinicians, and others, must appreciate how far the extent to which a child is an early or late maturer can modify the relationship between his size at any given age and the stature which he will eventually attain. They also need some method by which they can decide whether or not a small child is delayed in his maturation and by how much.

The many factors which influence the growth of normal healthy children and hence cause variation in the group must be understood if we are to recognize and correct any disturbance of growth which is pathological in origin.

This book is concerned with the nature, extent and causes of variation in the physical growth and development of children, whether they be healthy or are suffering from malfunction or disease. The recognition and differential diagnosis of growth disorders is discussed together with methods of treatment where appropriate. It is intended to be a practical book for the practical physician (or potential physician) who wishes to increase his understanding of the subject without becoming involved in too much jargon or unfamiliar statistical terminology.

July 1977   W. A. MARSHALL

Acknowledgements

My thanks are due to: Professor J. M. Tanner for introducing me, a long time ago, to the fascinating study of growth and for his helpful criticism of this manuscript; Dr D. B. Grant and Dr M. A. Preece for valuable advice on parts of the manuscript; Miss H. Davies, Miss S. Hedges and Miss G. Orrell for dealing with the practical difficulties of preparing the manuscript and illustrations and for many constructive suggestions they made in the process; to the publishers for their courtesy and cooperation and the many authors and publishers mentioned in the text who have kindly granted permission for me to reproduce material from their work.

Contents

Abbreviations Used in Text

ACTH	Adrenocorticotrophic hormone
B1, B2, etc.	Breast stages in girls
CNS	Central nervous system
DHA	Dehydroepiandrosterone
DNA	Deoxyribonucleic acid
DZ	Dizygotic
EEG	Electroencephalogram
FSH	Follicle stimulating hormone
FSHRH	Follicle stimulating hormone releasing hormone
G1, G2, etc.	Genital stages in boys
GnRH	Gonadotrophin releasing hormone
HGH	Human growth hormone
^{40}K	Potassium of atomic weight 40
LH	Luteinizing hormone
LHRH	Luteinizing hormone releasing hormone
M	Menarche
meq/kg	Milli-equivalents per kilogram
miu/ml	Micro international units per millilitre
MZ	Monozygotic
μm	Metres $\times$ 10^{-6}
nmol/l	Nanomoles per litre
PH1, PH2, etc.	Pubic hair stages
PHV	Peak height velocity
RUS	Radius ulna and short bones
RV	Residual volume
SD	Standard deviation
TLC	Total lung capacity
TSH	Thyroid stimulating hormone
TW2	Revized Tanner/Whitehouse method for estimating skeletal maturity
VC	Vital capacity

Methods of Studying Growth

INTRODUCTION

In clinical practice we have to decide whether or not our patients' growth deviates from the normal by comparing it with that of healthy children. If we wish to make a precise description of an abnormality we must have correspondingly precise information about the normal. Knowledge of any changes in growth pattern which occur between one decade and the next is valuable evidence about the effectiveness, or otherwise, of measures to improve or maintain the health and nutritional status of the community. Finally, we cannot formulate or test meaningful hypotheses about the mechanism concerned in the regulation of growth unless we have precise information about the events which are being regulated, that is, about the growth process itself. Thus, whether we are concerned with growth from the clinical point of view, in relation to community medicine, or as pure science; well-planned studies of normal children are the basis upon which we must build our knowledge.

METHODS OF DATA COLLECTION

Most growth studies are concerned with either
    (a) observing in detail the growth of individuals or
    (b) setting up "standards" giving the normal variation in a given parameter, e.g. stature, in a population of children at different ages.

The former aim is usually achieved most effectively by a longitudinal study and the latter by a cross-sectional one.

Longitudinal Studies

The best way to study the growth of any individual child is to measure him repeatedly. The collection of repeated measurements on the same individual, or group of individuals, constitutes a longitudinal study. Naturally the correct measurements must be taken and they must be accurate. The problems created by these two conditions will be considered later. We shall assume for the moment that we are dealing with accurate measurements of stature.

Stature and Stature Velocity. At the end of a longitudinal study we shall have a series of measurements for each individual at different ages and, by drawing a separate graph of stature against age for each subject, we shall have a reasonable description of his growth in stature. The graphs obtained in this way are "distance curves" (Fig. 1). If we had measured a number of normal individuals repeatedly in the course of a longitudinal study we should be able to plot a distance curve for each of them. All these curves would be similar in shape to the one shown in Fig. 1, which suggests that the child grew quickly during the first two years of

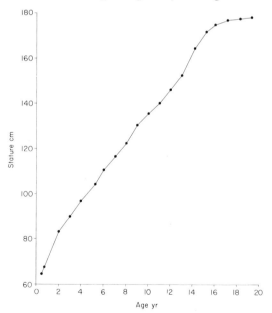

Fig. 1. Distance curve based on repeated measurements of the stature of a normal boy.

life but, after this, his stature increased fairly slowly and steadily until he was about 13 years old. He then experienced a sudden acceleration of growth, which we term the adolescent spurt. After the spurt, his growth slowed down until it finally stopped. This pattern of changes in speed of growth is followed by all normal children, although they differ in the exact speed at which they are growing at any given age. They also differ in the age at which major changes in growth rate, such as the adolescent spurt, take place.

The "distance curve" of a child's growth gives a very inadequate description of the growth pattern. It is not sufficient to say "he grew more quickly" or "he grew more slowly" as we have done in the previous paragraph. We want to know how quickly or how slowly. In other words, we want to know his exact growth rate (or "growth velocity") at each age. If we know this, we can plot a "velocity curve", similar to that shown in Fig. 2.

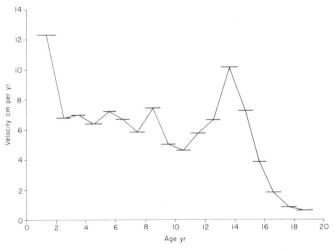

Fig. 2. Stature velocity based on the measurements shown in Fig. 1.

The term "growth velocity" or growth rate, refers to the increase in a given parameter (e.g. stature) in a specified period of time. Stature velocity is described in units of cm/yr, just as we talk about the speed of a motor car in miles/hour. To calculate the speed at which a vehicle is travelling we divide the distance travelled in miles by the time in hours or fractions of an hour. Similarly, we calculate growth velocity by dividing the distance grown (i.e. the difference between two successive measurements of stature, or whatever dimension we may be studying) by the time, in years, which has elapsed between the two measurements.

Thus, we might measure a child on his 10th birthday and again 13 weeks later, when he was 10·25 years old and discover that his stature had increased by 2 cm during that time. His growth rate during this three month period was therefore 2 cm divided by the time in years between the two measurements (i.e. 2 ÷ 0·25 yr) = 8 cm/yr. During the next few months he might grow at a quite different rate. Thus, although we measure growth rate in cm/yr, the speed may be calculated over any period of time, whether more or less than a year, just as we may calculate the average speed of a motor car in miles/hour over a few seconds or several hours. Indeed, the speed may change during the interval between the two measurements on which our calculation was based. We can calculate only the average growth velocity between the two successive measurements.

It would be very time-consuming to calculate growth velocities if we had to work out the time interval in months, weeks and days. Fortunately, this difficulty is easily overcome by the use of decimal dates (Table I). For example, if a child is measured on 3rd January (0·005 yr) and again on 19th May (0·378 yr) the time interval between the two measurements is 0·373 yr and the child's growth rate is calculated by dividing his increase in stature over this period by 0·373 yr. The answer is in cm/yr. For practical purposes we usually correct the time intervals to two decimal places, i.e. to the nearest 3·65 days. The third decimal place represents less than half a day.

We can construct a growth velocity curve for any individual who has been measured repeatedly if we calculate his velocity between successive pairs of measurements. The velocities are usually plotted as horizontal lines extending from the age at the first measurement to the age at the second measurement, as shown on the x-axis. If we repeat the calculations for each pair of measurements from birth to maturity and plot the results we shall obtain a curve similar to Fig. 2, which is based on measurements of an actual child. This velocity curve describes the child's growth much more clearly than the distance curve (Fig. 1) and is typical of normal children. It shows that the subject was growing at an average rate of 12 cm/yr from the age of about six months to two years (just after birth the rate may have been nearly 20 cm/yr). From this time the velocity fluctuated, with a general downward trend, reaching a minimum of 4 or 5 cm/yr just before the adolescent spurt began. During the spurt, a maximal velocity of 10 cm/yr was reached, but was followed by a marked deceleration. The maximal velocity achieved during the adolescent spurt is termed "peak height velocity" (PHV) and is an important "landmark" in the growth of all normal children. From a velocity curve we can see the age at which the child

TABLE I

Calendar dates expressed as decimals

	1 Jan.	2 Feb.	3 Mar.	4 Apr.	5 May	6 June	7 July	8 Aug.	9 Sep.	10 Oct.	11 Nov.	12 Dec.
1	000	085	162	247	329	414	496	581	666	748	833	915
2	003	088	164	249	332	416	499	584	668	751	836	918
3	005	090	167	252	334	419	501	586	671	753	838	921
4	008	093	170	255	337	422	504	589	674	756	841	923
5	011	096	173	258	340	425	507	592	677	759	844	926
6	014	099	175	260	342	427	510	595	679	762	847	929
7	016	101	178	263	345	430	512	597	682	764	849	932
8	019	104	181	266	348	433	515	600	685	767	852	934
9	022	107	184	268	351	436	518	603	688	770	855	937
10	025	110	186	271	353	438	521	605	690	773	858	940
11	027	112	189	274	356	441	523	608	693	775	860	942
12	030	115	192	277	359	444	526	611	696	778	863	945
13	033	118	195	279	362	447	529	614	699	781	866	948
14	036	121	197	282	364	449	532	616	701	784	868	951
15	038	123	200	285	367	452	534	619	704	786	871	953
16	041	126	203	288	370	455	537	622	707	789	874	956
17	044	129	205	290	373	458	540	625	710	792	877	959
18	047	132	208	293	375	460	542	627	712	795	879	962
19	049	134	211	296	378	463	545	630	715	797	882	964
20	052	137	214	299	381	466	548	633	718	800	885	967
21	055	140	216	301	384	468	551	636	721	803	888	970
22	058	142	219	304	386	471	553	638	723	805	890	973
23	060	145	222	307	389	474	556	641	726	808	893	975
24	063	148	225	310	392	477	559	644	729	811	896	978
25	066	151	227	312	395	479	562	647	731	814	899	981
26	068	153	230	315	397	482	564	649	734	816	901	984
27	071	156	233	318	400	485	567	652	737	819	904	986
28	074	159	236	321	403	488	570	655	740	822	907	989
29	077		238	323	405	490	573	658	742	825	910	992
30	079		241	326	408	493	575	660	745	827	912	995
31	082		244		411		578	663		830		997

Jan.	Feb.	Mar.	Apr.	May	June	July	Aug.	Sep.	Oct.	Nov.	Dec.
1	2	3	4	5	6	7	8	9	10	11	12

attained PHV as well as its actual value in cm/yr. This kind of information can be obtained only from repeated measurements of the same individual. It cannot be obtained by measuring different individuals at each age, even if a very large number are studied.

When we have studied several individuals longitudinally, it is easy to examine the growth curve for each of them but, if we wish to combine them as a group, we have a much more difficult problem.

Figures 3a and 3b show the distance and velocity curves of five children, all of whom have normal statures and growth rates. However, as we should find in any group of normal children, they do not all experience the adolescent spurt at the same age. If we were to take the average of their statures at each age, we should obtain the curve represented by the interrupted line in Fig. 3a. Although this is a true representation of the average heights of the children, it does not describe the growth of a "typical" child or, indeed, of any child. The "adolescent spurt" indicated by this curve is not nearly as steep as it is in any individual and lasts for a much longer time.

The same argument applies to our collection of velocity curves where the average (again shown by an interrupted curve) suggests that the adolescent spurt is more prolonged in time but does not reach nearly as great a maximal velocity as it actually does in any individual.

One simple way of overcoming this difficulty, which is due to the spurt occurring at different ages in different subjects, is to eliminate age completely from our graph. Instead of taking birth as our zero point we might take a distinct point on each curve, such as the peak of the adolescent growth spurt (PHV). The time scale would then be plotted in years before and after PHV and the result is shown in Fig. 4a, where the interrupted line constructed by joining the average velocities at each point on the time scale is a fair representation of what actually happens in a typical individual. Then we could, if we wished, replot our five "distance curves" on a similar axis (Fig. 4b) and construct a much more meaningful "average distance curve".

Curve Fitting. A more precise approach to longitudinal data demands mathematical curve fitting procedures. A fitted curve is essentially a shorthand way of describing the growth process and fitting the curve is an important step in dealing with some research problems. However, curve fitting does not enter into clinical work and details of the method are beyond the scope of this book. The basic principles are, however, simple. The simplest form of curve is a straight line and is described by the equation

$$y = bx + c$$

where b is a constant indicating the slope of the line and c is a constant representing the value of y at which the line crosses the y-axis (Fig. 5), i.e. when $x = 0$. If it were possible to describe growth in stature by a straight line, with stature on the y-axis and age on the x-axis, b would be the rate of growth and c would be the length of the child at birth.

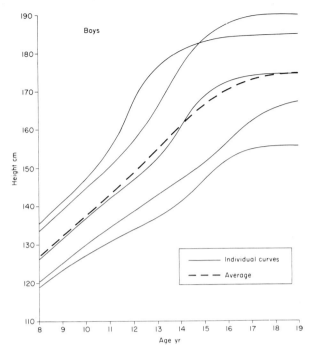

Fig. 3a. Growth in stature of five boys (distance curves). The interrupted line indicates the mean stature of the boys at each age.

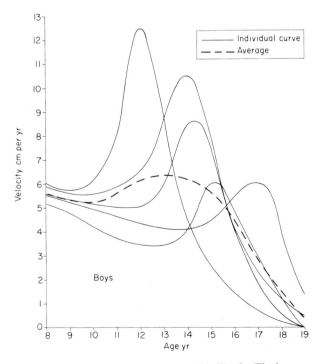

Fig. 3b. Stature velocity curves of the boys represented in Fig. 3a. The interrupted line shows the mean velocity of the boys at each age.

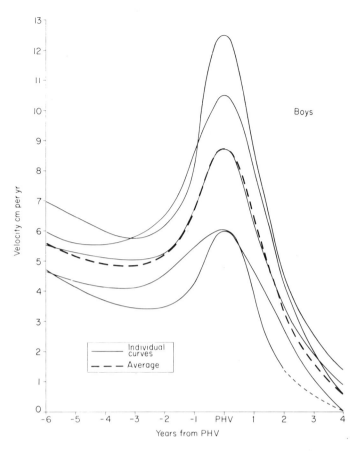

Fig. 4a. The velocity curves of Fig. 3b plotted in relation to peak height velocity. The interrupted line shows the mean for the group.

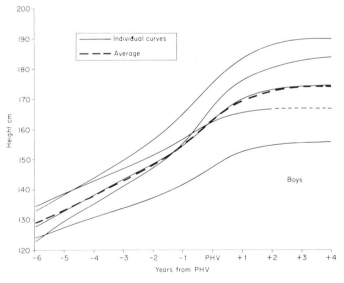

Fig. 4b. The distance curves of Fig. 3a plotted in relation to peak height velocity. The interrupted line shows the mean for the group.

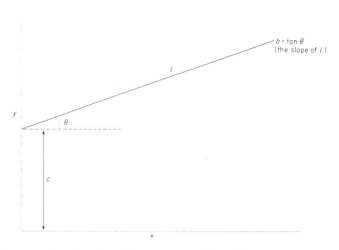

Fig. 5. Diagrammatic explanation of the parameters "*b*" and "*c*" in the equation $y = bx + c$ describing a straight line *l*.

However, most growth processes cannot be described by straight lines and we have to use equations with more constants (usually raising variables to higher powers) to represent curves with more complex shapes. This can only be done usefully with data from longitudinal studies. The usual procedure is to plot a "distance" graph of the measurements of the chosen parameter (e.g. stature) for each child and then decide what shape of mathematically fitted curve will fit them most accurately and describe them most usefully. The curve should be one represented by an equation whose constants have some real biological meaning (as for example *b* would represent the growth rate if we were to fit a straight line).

The curve represented by this equation would then be fitted to the data for each child in turn. The fitting process involves calculating the constants, which would have different numerical values for each child. In order to obtain a curve which would describe the group of children we could take the mean value of the constants. Again, taking the simple example of a straight line, the mean value of *b* would be the average growth rate and the mean value of *c* would be the mean length at birth. A curve calculated in this way is called a "mean constant curve". This, in most cases is quite different from a "mean curve" which would be obtained by taking the mean value of the measurements at each age and then fitting the curve. In the case of a straight line, the "mean" and "mean constant" curves are identical but this is seldom true of more complex curves.

The growth in stature of a single adolescent could be described quite well by the "S" shaped Gompertz curve which has the equation

$$Y = P + K \exp[-\exp(a - bt)]$$

where Y = stature; t = age; P = lower asymptote (i.e. stature at the beginning of the adolescent spurt which is described by the curve); K = gain in stature during adolescence, i.e. difference between upper and lower asymptote. The final adult stature of the individual is therefore $P + K$: a is a constant integration and b is a constant representing the rate at which the proportion $(Y - P)/K$ is increasing to equal powers of itself. The product bKe^{-1} represents the maximum rate of growth attained, i.e. peak height velocity.

The use of the Gompertz curve in describing growth during adolescence is discussed in greater detail by Deming (1957) and Marubini *et al.* (1972). Marubini *et al.* found that the Logistic curve which is similar in shape but with the formula

$$Y = P + K/[1 + \exp(a - bt)]$$

(where symbols have the same meaning as in the Gompertz curve) fits the data slightly better. They recommend it as the best equation fitting growth data on skeletal dimensions at adolescence.

In order to describe the adolescent spurt in a group of subjects we should fit a Logistic curve to the data for each individual, i.e. calculate the values of the constants for each subject. The mean values of the constants could then be used to plot a mean constant curve. It would give a quite erroneous picture if we were to calculate a curve based on the mean values of the measurements at each age.

It is usually most convenient to calculate velocity curves by differentiation of the equation of a "distance curve" fitted to the original measurements.

Pros and Cons of Longitudinal Studies. Longitudinal studies have important advantages and disadvantages. The main advantages are that they reveal accurately the growth patterns of individuals; enable us to study changes in speed of growth; enable us to study any sequence of events such as the eruption of the teeth or the development of the secondary sex characteristics. For example, the average time which elapses between the beginning of breast development in an adolescent girl and the occurrence of her first menstrual period is about two and a half years. In some individuals, however, this interval is less than one year while in others it is more than five. Information of this kind can be obtained only by longitudinal studies.

The main disadvantages of longitudinal studies are, firstly, that they are time consuming. A study of the complete growth of a group of children cannot be completed in less than 20 years. During this time many of the subjects will withdraw from the study for various reasons. For some purposes, of course, it may be sufficient to carry out a longitudinal study over only a limited number of years. Secondly, it is impossible to carry out a longitudinal study on a sample sufficiently large to be truly representative of the population. The expense of doing so would be prohibitive.

For some purposes the longitudinal method is not the most efficient way of collecting data and a cross-sectional study is more appropriate.

Cross-sectional Studies

Cross-sectional studies are those in which a group of children is measured at each stage but no individual is measured more than once. For example, we might measure the statures of a thousand 5-year-old boys, a different thousand aged 7 and so on. This is the most effective method of estimating the mean value of any given measurement, e.g. stature, in children of different age groups, and also of measuring the variation about this mean. Population "standards" and "growth charts" for clinical use are based very largely on cross-sectional data, although they may be modified in the light of information obtained by longitudinal studies.

A longitudinal study is less satisfactory than a cross-sectional one for estimating the population mean at successive ages. This is due to the fact that the samples at each age in a longitudinal study are not independent of each other (i.e. they are the same children). A cross-sectional study is therefore the correct method of setting up population standards describing the mean and variation in height, weight or any other parameter in children at different ages. It is possible, within quite a short time, to measure a large and representative sample of children of each age group.

However, as we have seen above, a curve obtained by plotting the means at each age, as estimated by cross-sectional study, will not represent correctly the shape of the growth curve of any individual. The distortion is greatest at those ages when some individuals are more advanced than others in their progress through the adolescent spurt. Furthermore, a cross-sectional study will not give us useful information about the variations in rate of growth of the children in the population as this can only be obtained by measuring each child at least twice.

In order to create growth standards which describe the variation in growth velocity amongst children at each age, the most satisfactory approach is to carry out a cross-sectional study with a large number of children at each age and then repeat the whole study one year later. It is then possible to calculate each child's growth velocity over one year. Taking this value for each individual, we can calculate the mean and variance of the velocity for each age group. The height and weight velocity standards shown in the next chapter were calculated in this way although the basic data were somewhat different. These standards do not, of course, provide a description of any individual's velocity curve but lead to the situation already illustrated in Fig. 3b. They describe correctly the mean and range of variation in velocity at each age separately. The pattern of change with age in individuals can be determined only by longitudinal studies.

Mixed Longitudinal Studies

Sometimes, for practical reasons, a study is carried out in which some subjects are measured repeatedly over long periods, some over short periods and some perhaps only once. This is a mixed longitudinal study and can provide very useful information but requires special statistical methods to interpret the data.

In conclusion, it is wrong to say that longitudinal studies are better than cross-sectional ones, or vice versa. Each has its proper place. The important thing is to ensure that the type of study is appropriate to the questions which are being asked and the kind of conclusion the observer hopes to draw. When we are reading a report, we must satisfy ourselves that the conclusions that have been drawn are justified by the design of the study on which they are based.

THE BASIC MEASUREMENTS

For clinical purposes, we can obtain most of the information we require about a child's growth from the measurements of stature and sitting height. If we also want to know whether the child is becoming fatter or thinner we should measure the thickness of skin and subcutaneous fat with skin calipers.

Weight

Although weight is a widely used measurement, it is a very unsatisfactory one. An increase in weight might be due to growth but, on the other hand, it might be due mainly to an increase in the fat or water content of the body. Alternatively, quite adequate growth may not be accompanied by a significant increase in weight, if fat is lost at the same time. Nevertheless, a very abnormal weight, or failure to gain weight at a satisfactory rate over a long period, indicates that something is wrong and is a signal for further investigation of the child's health and/or diet. Routine weighing, particularly of babies, therefore has some value and is a useful method of supervizing the general health and nutrition of children when time and facilities are limited.

Unfortunately, weight is still frequently used as an index of growth when the above strictures do not apply and other measures such as length or stature could be used to obtain more precise information. However, because it is easy to weigh children and because mothers throughout most of the world expect this to be done, the practice will no doubt continue. Therefore, in interpreting weight, the following points must be remembered. (i) A child who is very light as compared with others of his age may be abnormally small or abnormally thin or both. (ii) If he is not gaining weight at the expected rate for his age he may be growing too slowly, or he might be growing at a very satisfactory rate and losing fat. If he were too fat in the first place this would be a good thing. (iii) A child who is unusually heavy for his age might be too fat or he might be just a big child. (iv) If he is gaining weight very rapidly he might be gaining too much fat, or on the other hand, he might just be growing quickly without tendency to become obese.

Clearly then, weight is only a very approximate guide to the child's growth and is obviously even less reliable if the technique is not standardized. The child should be nude or wearing only very light clothing. Ideally the bowels and bladder should be evacuated and, if the same child is to be measured repeatedly, this should be done at approximately the same time of day on each occasion.

Stature

The significance of changes in a child's weight, whether they are apparently too big or too small, can be determined only by taking other measurements, of which the most important is stature, or supine length in the child who is too young to stand.

Stature must be measured accurately, otherwise it is impossible to make a reliable estimate of the child's rate of growth between successive measurements. This apparently obvious statement clearly needs emphasis as many of the measurements of stature taken in schools, doctors' surgeries and hospitals are so inaccurate as to be not only of little value but totally misleading. Errors of 3 to 4 cm are not uncommon whereas, when a correct technique is used, the error should very rarely exceed 3 mm. We must remember that the growth of a healthy pre-adolescent child may be in the region of 6 cm/yr or even less. If we measure him on two occasions with an interval of six months between them he will have grown only 3 cm. This amount of growth cannot be measured satisfactorily if the error of the individual measurements exceeds 2 or 3 mm. A positive error of 1·5 cm on the first occasion and a negative one of the same magnitude on the second would suggest that he had not grown at all. On the other hand, if the first error were negative and the second positive, he would appear to have grown 6 cm in six months, or at a rate of 12 cm/yr. We should then have to seek an explanation for his apparently abnormally rapid growth.

Sometimes the error is inherent in the measuring instrument. This instrument may consist of a rod which is supposed to be vertical, but in fact is sufficiently flexible to enable it to bend far from vertical during use. A horizontal bar should be attached at right-angles so that it can move up and down the rod, always at the same angle. Frequently, however, this bar does not remain consistently at right-angles to the rod. Such instruments are commonly used and cannot give a true measurement even if the technique for positioning the child and reading the measurement is perfect.

In addition, the child may be positioned in such a way that the measurement is not taken to the top of the head, or even to the same part of the head on repeated occasions. Sometimes children are even measured with their shoes on.

For clinical work, children must be measured with an accurate instrument and in a standard posture. The basic components of an instrument for measuring stature are: (i) a firm horizontal surface on which the subject stands; (ii) a rigid vertical surface which can be brought into contact with his back; (iii) another horizontal surface (as distinct from a narrow rod) which can move up and down the vertical one, is always at right-angles to it, and can be brought into contact with the top of the child's head; (iv) a means of measuring the distance between the two horizontal surfaces.

An instrument such as the Harpenden Stadiometer (Fig. 6) is ideal but if this is not available, a non-rigid instrument of the type mentioned above is not a satisfactory alternative. It is better to use the floor, the wall (with a measuring scale attached to it) and a block of wood which may be moved up and down against the wall at right-angles to it. The surface which comes into contact with the head should be at least 15 cm square and a similar area at right-angles to this should be in contact with the wall. A useful refinement would be to fit the block of wood, which functions as a head-board, to runners and attach it to counterweights over pulleys. If this is not done the head-board has to be held against the wall and two people are required to take the measurements; one to hold the head-board and the other to hold the child's head and take the reading.

The child must have his socks and shoes removed, as loose socks may conceal the fact that he is raising his heels from the ground while he is being measured. The observer asks him to stand with his heels, scapulae

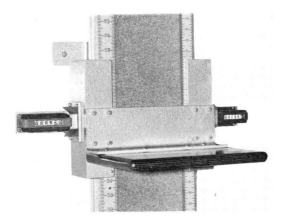

Fig. 6. The Harpenden Stadiometer.

and buttocks touching the vertical surface and encourages him to relax as much as possible. The observer positions the child's head so that the lower borders of the orbits are in the same horizontal plane as the external auditory meati, the so-called "Frankfurt plane", and exerts gentle upward pressure on the mastoid processes (Fig. 7) while giving the child verbal encouragement to "make himself as tall as possible". This upward pressure extends the child to his full height and helps to correct any temporary variation in posture. Care must be taken to ensure that the child does not raise his heels from the ground. Young children very often do this and it may be helpful to ask them to "wiggle their toes", i.e. to raise the toes from the ground and move them. While they are doing this they find it extremely difficult to raise their heels from the ground. If this stratagem is not successful, the child's mother or an assistant must hold his heels on the floor. The measurement is read to the last completed mm, i.e. it is not "corrected up" if it appears to be nearer to the next mm.

Stature is the best measure of the child's overall size but gives us no information about the relationship between the length of the lower limbs and that of the trunk. It is important that this relationship should be studied in normal children because it varies between populations and is altered in some disorders of growth. It is very difficult to obtain accurate measurements of the lower limb without using X-rays, but for many purposes, including clinical practice, it is quite satisfactory to study the relationship between sitting height and either stature or sub-ischial length (stature minus sitting height).

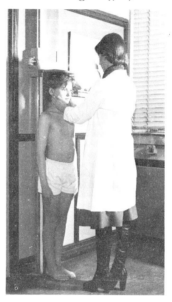

Fig. 7. The measurement of stature. Note the position of the subject's head and the observer's hands as they exert upward pressure on the mastoid processes.

Sitting Height

Sitting height is measured with the subject sitting on a table. The feet are supported so that the distal tendons above and beyond the knee are clear of the table by about three centimetres. The hands are relaxed on the thighs. A Harpenden anthropometer (see Fig. 8) with an extension fitted and the blade nearest the extension removed, is held vertically in the midline of the subject's back, but not touching it. The head is positioned in the Frankfurt plane, as for stature, and gentle upward pressure is applied to it. The subject is told to sit upright and make himself as tall as possible. Some children tend to lift their buttocks off the table while they are being measured. This can be largely avoided by supporting the feet so that the biceps femoris tendons are 3 cm clear of the table, as in Fig. 8. Other specially designed instruments may be

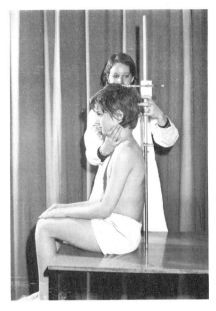

Fig. 8. The measurement of sitting height using the Harpenden Anthropometer. Note the observer's hands exerting gentle upward pressure to position the subject's head.

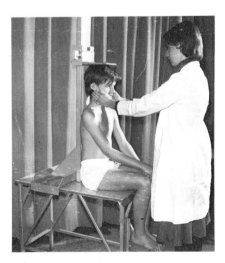

Fig. 9. The measurement of sitting height using the Harpenden Sitting Height Table.

used (Fig. 9) or the instrument normally used to measure stature may be adapted by putting a narrow table in front of it.

The Harpenden anthropometer may be used to take other measurements such as shoulder and hip widths and the lengths of the upper arm, forearm and leg. Unfortunately, there is no satisfactory method of measuring the length of the thigh with anthropometric instruments, owing to the lack of a bony point near the upper end of the femur which can be accurately palpated in all subjects. These measurements, however, are usually required only in highly specialized work and need not be discussed in detail here.

Skinfolds

When we want to know if a child is gaining or losing fat, his weight helps us very little. If we knew how much his height had increased over a period of time, we might be able to make a subjective judgement as to whether or not the weight gain over the same period was excessive or insufficient in relation to the growth in stature. However, it would be much more satisfactory if we could make a more direct measurement of change in the amount of fat.

For clinical purposes we need a relatively simple technique by which we can tell whether the amount of subcutaneous fat is increasing or decreasing. The techniques for estimating body fat from measurements such as body density, as discussed in Chapter 7, are too complicated for widespread use, and measurements of skinfold thickness are more appropriate.

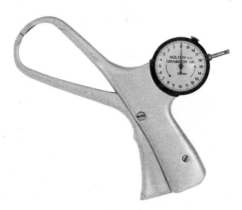

Fig. 10. The Holtain Skinfold Caliper.

In many parts of the body the skin and subcutaneous tissues are only loosely attached to underlying structures and can be picked up between the thumb and forefinger as a fold. The thickness of this fold can be measured between the jaws of a caliper (Fig. 10). As the thickness of the skin itself is more or less constant, variations in skinfold thickness are essentially due to differences in the amount of subcutaneous fat.

Clearly the thickness of any fold of soft tissue is partially dependent upon the pressure exerted on it. Therefore the caliper must be designed so that the pressure between its jaws does not change whether they are close together or far apart. By international agreement all skinfold calipers should exert a constant pressure of 10 g/mm². The Harpenden caliper and the Holtain caliper developed from it (see Fig. 10) are the best available.

The skinfold is measured by picking up a fold of skin and sub-cutaneous tissue between the observer's forefinger and thumb, which are initially placed about 2 cm apart on the skin and then brought together to pinch the fold away from the underlying muscle (Fig. 11).

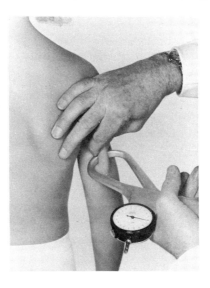

Fig. 11. Measuring the triceps skinfold.

The jaws of the caliper are applied to the skinfold about 2 cm below the fingers. The right hand then relaxes its grip on the handle so that the jaws can exert their full pressure. The dial of the caliper is calibrated at intervals of 0·2 mm but the measurement can reasonably be estimated to the nearest 0·1 mm. The left hand continues to pinch the fold throughout the measurement. This technique usually results in a stable reading up to values of 20 mm but at a higher value the measurement registered on the dial sometimes decreases. A firmer grip on the left hand may prevent this but, if not, the reading should be taken two seconds after the caliper is applied. The skinfold thickness is read to the nearest completed 0·1 and not to the one above, even if it appears to have nearly reached it.

During growth, the amount of subcutaneous fat deposited on the limbs is often different from that on the trunk. For this reason it is advisable to take fat measurements on both limb and trunk sites. The triceps and subscapular sites are most frequently used and it is usually quite easy to pick up the skinfold "cleanly". In some girls, and obese children of either sex, the fold cannot be adequately picked up and a valid measurement is not possible.

The triceps skinfold is measured over the posterior surface of the left triceps muscle on a vertical line passing upwards from the olecranon, with the arm hanging relaxed at the side. The observer palpates the tips of the acromion process and the olecranon and marks a point on the skin half-way between them. The skinfold is picked up by placing the fingers slightly above this mark and the caliper jaws are applied at the marked level. It is important that the measurement is made on the correct vertical line on the back of the arm, as different values are obtained at sites lateral or medial to this.

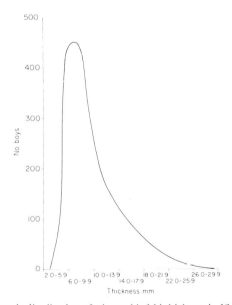

Fig. 12. Schematic distribution of triceps skinfold thickness in 12-year old boys.

The subscapular skinfold is picked up just below the angle of the left scapula by the observer's thumb and forefinger which are brought down the lateral and medial borders of the bone, until they meet. The fold itself may be in a vertical line or slightly inclined in the natural cleavage line of the skin.

Skinfold measurements do not have the same accuracy as, for example, the measurement of stature, but a trained observer should duplicate his readings within $\pm 5\%$ in two-thirds or more of all repeated measurements (Edwards *et al.*, 1955). Differences between observers may be much greater than this unless great care is taken in training them together and unless the relationships between their readings are frequently checked.

If skinfold thicknesses are studied in a population, the frequency distribution is found to be skewed as in Fig. 12. Most of the widely used methods of statistical analyses are invalid when applied to skewed distributions and it is therefore an advantage if the skewness can be minimized by a simple mathematical transformation. The most suitable transform for triceps and subscapular skinfolds in both sexes is

$$\text{skinfold transform} = 100 \times \log_{10} (\text{reading in mm} - 1 \cdot 8)$$

i.e. take the caliper reading in units of $0 \cdot 1$ mm and subtract $1 \cdot 8$ mm. Take the logarithm base 10 of the answer and multiply by 100. A table of the transformed skinfold thicknesses is given by Edwards *et al.* (1955). If the measurements are plotted on the standard skinfold charts published by Tanner and Whitehouse (1975) shown in Figs 13 and 14, it is not necessary to calculate the transform as the adjustment is made by the scale on the chart. However, if a statistical comparison is to be made between groups of children, the transform of each skinfold reading should be calculated before proceeding to further statistical tests.

RELATIONSHIP BETWEEN TWO PARAMETERS

When we have measured two parameters, such as stature and sitting height, the method of expressing the relationship between them presents a problem. In the past, it was a common practice to divide one parameter by the other to make a ratio e.g. sitting height/stature. This procedure has the disadvantage that it discards the information that we have about the absolute values of the measurements. If the ratio is high, we do not know if this is due to a high sitting height or a low stature. Also, the simple use of ratios does not tell us whether their values alter in normal children with increasing age and overall size which, in fact, they do. For example, in an infant whose sitting height was 50 cm and

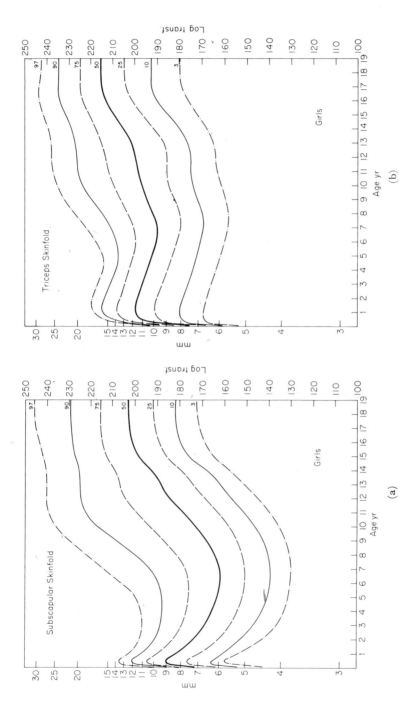

Fig. 13a and b. Centiles of skinfold thickness – girls. Reproduced from Tanner and Whitehouse (1975) with permission.

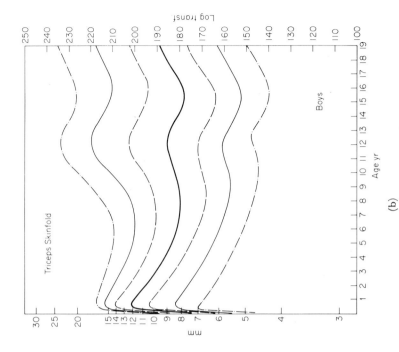

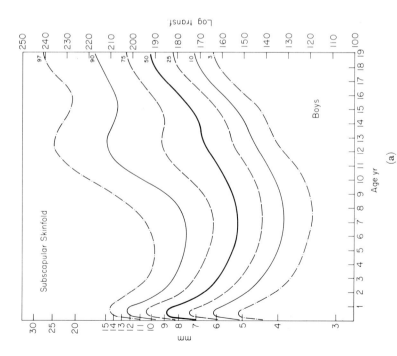

Fig. 14a and b. Centiles of skinfold thickness – boys. Reproduced from Tanner and Whitehouse (1975) with permission.

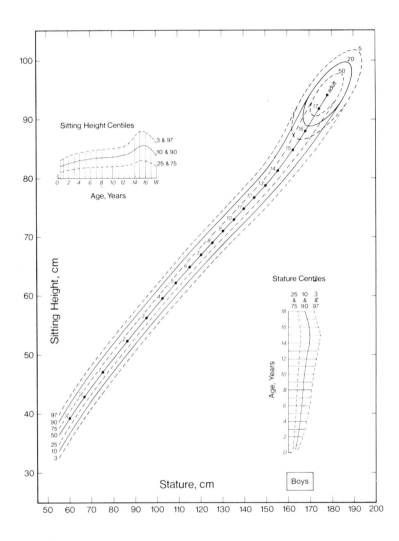

Fig. 15. Relationship between sitting height and stature in boys. Reproduced by kind permission of Professor J. M. Tanner.

whose stature was 80 cm, the resulting sitting height/stature ratio of 0·62 would be entirely normal. However, in an adolescent 150 cm tall, the same ratio would imply a sitting height of 93 cm which would be grossly abnormal in a person of this size. The legs would be extremely short in relation to the trunk.

A more satisfactory way of relating two parameters, which overcomes

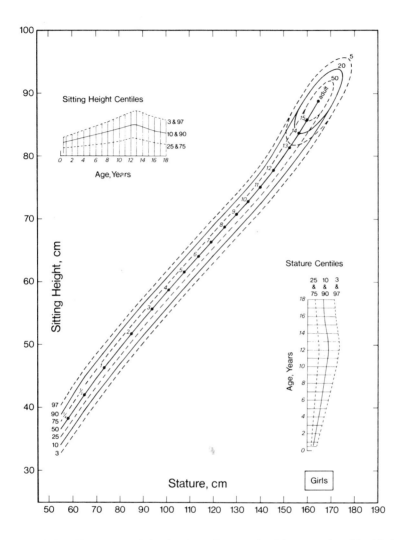

Fig. 16. Relationship between sitting height and stature in girls. Reproduced by kind per mission of Professor J. M. Tanner.

the above difficulties, is simply to plot one measurement against the other. If we had carried out a cross-sectional study in which we measured stature and sitting height in a large number of children, we could classify them in order of their stature and then make a graph, with stature as the x-axis and sitting height as the y-axis, and plot the measurements for each child. Alternatively, we might divide the sample of children into groups according to stature then work out the mean value of sitting height for each stature class and plot this. We might also calculate some measure of the variation in sitting height in each given stature group. The charts in Figs 15 and 16 were constructed in this way although rather complicated statistical procedures, beyond the scope of this book, were used to estimate the mean values and the variation about them. The variation is expressed as centiles, the interpretation of which is discussed in Chapter 2. This is the most satisfactory method of describing the relationship between any two measurements in children. In specialized work the method may be complicated or refined in various ways but the underlying principle is the same. It should be noted, however, that the slope of the line obtained when one measurement is plotted against another within a single age group is not necessarily the same as that of the line which would be obtained if a number of ages were combined.

2

Variations in the Growth of Normal Children

CENTILES AS A MEASURE OF VARIATION

The variation in a given measurement, e.g. stature or birth weight, in children of any age is most conveniently described in terms of centiles. If a large sample of children in a single age group is measured, 50% of them will be found to have a stature below a certain value. This value is the 50th centile. Only 3% have statures below another lower value which we therefore define as the third centile. At the other extreme the statures of only 3% of subjects are above the 97th centile. Other centiles may be similarly defined.

Birth Weight Centiles

Sometimes a child's birth weight is the only information that we can obtain about his intra-uterine growth. Mothers usually know the birth weights of their children but not their lengths. Usually a mother will also know if the baby was "early" or "late" in relation to its expected date of delivery. If the baby is still very young she may even remember the date of her last menstrual period. From this information we can work out the "gestational" or, to be more precise, the post-menstrual, age of the baby at birth. The post-menstrual age is only an approximate indication of the true gestational age. It is subject to errors resulting from variations in the length of the menstrual cycle; in time of ovulation within the cycle and in time of conception in relation to ovulation. Further error may result from inaccurate recall of the date of the last menstrual period or from vaginal bleeding in early pregnancy.

Centile charts (Tanner and Thomson, 1970) are available showing the variation in birth weight at different post-menstrual ages (Figs 17 and 18). These, of necessity, are based on cross-sectional data and describe only the variation in the weights of babies who are actually born at a given post-menstrual age. Thus the centiles for babies born at 36 weeks may not accurately describe the variation in weight (at 36 weeks) of foetuses which remain *in utero* until term. However, we can take it that a baby whose birth weight is below the 3rd centile for its gestational age is abnormally small.

It is important to distinguish between a child with a birth weight which is low in comparison with full term babies, but normal for the child's own gestational age, and an infant whose birth weight is low, even when its gestational age is taken into account. The former child was born after a short gestation, but its growth up to birth was normal. Such children follow a normal pattern of growth throughout childhood and reach normal adult height. The "small for gestational age" or "small for dates" baby on the other hand frequently remains small throughout childhood and becomes a small adult.

It should be noted that the centiles for first born babies are lower than those which describe the variation in birth weight of later children in the family. Also, there is a tendency for bigger mothers to have bigger babies, although, of course, many small women have had big babies. The 3rd centile for the babies of tall mothers is higher than that for all babies. A certain amount should therefore be subtracted from the birth weight of a tall mother's baby before it is plotted on the chart. Similarly, something should be added to the birth weight if the mother is small. These amounts may be determined from the diagram above the centile charts in Figs 17 and 18.

The range of birth weights amongst babies of a given gestational age is considerable and a heavy baby at, for example, 36 weeks, may be much heavier than a small full-term baby. Thus weight is not an indication of gestational age and there are no grounds for describing a baby as "premature" because it has a low birth weight. If the length of gestation is known it can be classified as either "normal" or "small" for gestational age. It is current practice to describe babies born before 37 weeks as "preterm"; those born between 37 and 42 weeks as "term" and later births as "post-term".

TABLE II

Birth length at different gestational ages

(Based on data from Usher and McLean, 1974.)

Gestation (weeks)	Crown – Heel Length (cm) Centiles		
	3rd	50th	97th
25	31·8	34·6	37·4
26	32·8	35·6	38·4
27	33·7	36·6	39·5
28	34·7	37·6	40·5
29	35·8	38·8	41·8
30	36·8	39·9	43·0
31	38·0	41·1	44·2
32	39·2	42·4	45·6
33	40·5	43·7	46·9
34	41·7	45·0	48·3
35	42·9	46·2	49·5
36	44·0	47·4	50·8
37	45·2	48·6	52·0
38	46·3	49·8	53·3
39	47·2	50·7	54·2
40	47·6	51·2	54·8
41	48·1	51·7	55·3

Birth Length Centiles

The length of babies at a given gestational age also varies considerably as shown by a study carried out by Usher and McLean (1969) of 300 Canadian babies of European descent and of mixed national and socioeconomic backgrounds (see Table II).

Unfortunately, because it is the traditional practice to weigh babies at birth and not to measure them, there is very little information on birth lengths in most populations. More babies are now being measured at birth and it is to be hoped that this practice will spread so that a good record of normal data can be established. If, at the same time, mothers are encouraged to remember their babies' lengths, the diagnosis of intrauterine growth retardation will become much easier, even when we meet it in the form of short stature in later childhood.

Stature Centiles

If we measure a large number of different children at each age, i.e. carry out a cross-sectional study, we can calculate the centiles for stature

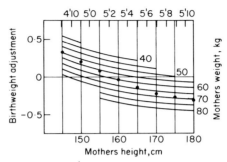

Adjustment for mother's height and mid - pregnancy weight to be added
or subtracted from birthweight. Scale as in chart below. If weight
unknown, use ● points.

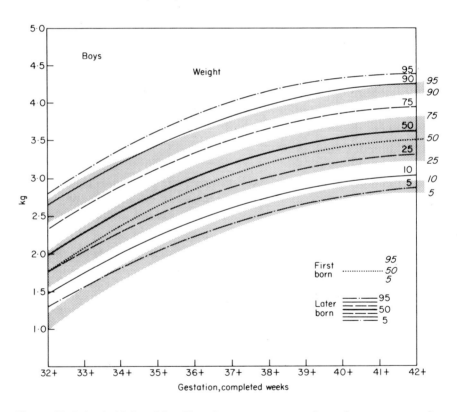

Fig. 17. Variation in birth weight of boys born at postmenstrual ages from 32 to 42 weeks, allowing for maternal height and weight. Reproduced from Tanner and Thomson (1970) with permission.

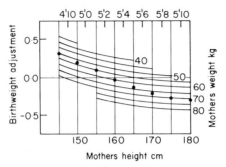

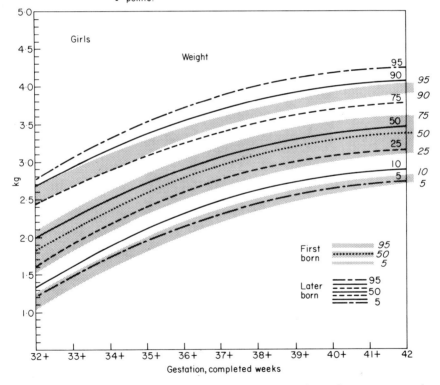

Fig. 18. Variation in birth weight of girls born at postmenstrual ages from 32 to 42 weeks allowing for maternal height and weight. Reproduced from Tanner and Thomson (1970) with permission.

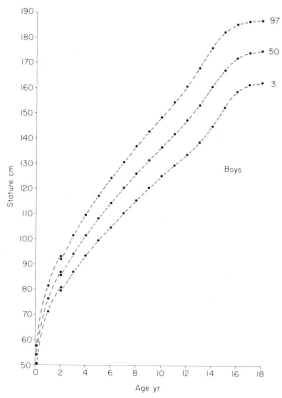

Fig. 19. Chart showing the 3rd, 50th and 97th centiles for stature based on separate samples of boys at each year of age after 2 years and supine length at earlier ages.

at each age (Fig. 19). If we plot these values and join them we have a "centile chart" from which we can estimate the centiles at any inter-mediate age. The actual values of the stature centiles for British children at different ages are shown in Table III.

A centile chart based on cross-sectional data consists of a series of lines which are similar, but not identical, to the growth curves of individual children. Up to the age of 8, the growth curves of many individuals would be more or less parallel to one of these centile lines, but, after this age, the centile lines do not illustrate the shape of the growth curve for any individual child.

This situation arises because the adolescent growth spurt (see page 38) occurs at different ages in different individuals, so that in a group of 12-year-old children for example, the growth of some would have begun to accelerate while others would still be growing at a pre-adolescent rate. As we have seen in the previous chapter, only longitudinal data

TABLE III

Centiles for stature (cross-sectional type)

(Based on data from Tanner *et al.*, 1966.)

Age (yr)	Boys			Girls		
	3rd	50th centiles (cm)	97th	3rd	50th centiles (cm)	97th
2·0	79·7	85·9	92·1	78·4	84·6	90·8
3·0	87·0	94·2	101·4	85·7	93·0	100·2
4·0	93·5	101·6	109·7	92·3	100·4	108·5
5·0	99·4	108·3	117·2	98·2	107·2	116·1
6·0	104·9	114·6	124·3	103·8	113·4	123·1
7·0	110·3	120·5	130·8	109·1	119·3	129·6
8·0	115·4	126·2	137·0	114·2	125·0	125·8
9·0	120·4	131·6	142·9	119·3	130·6	141·9
10·0	125·1	136·8	148·5	124·5	136·4	148·3
11·0	129·4	141·9	154·4	129·5	142·7	155·8
12·0	133·7	147·3	160·9	135·0	149·3	163·6
13·0	138·7	153·4	168·2	142·6	155·5	168·5
14·0	145·0	160·7	176·2	147·6	159·6	171·6
15·0	152·3	167·3	182·4	150·3	161·7	173·2
16·0	158·9	172·2	185·5	150·9	162·2	173·5
17·0	161·7	174·3	186·8			
18·0	162·2	174·7	187·2			

will correctly describe the growth spurt in an individual. The curve which would be obtained by plotting repeated measurements of any individual's stature against age during his adolescent spurt would be steeper than a curve obtained by joining the average (50th centile) values calculated from samples of different children at each chronological age.

In order to make a chart which bears a closer relationship to the shapes of the growth curves of actual children, we must eliminate the variation in timing of the adolescent spurt and draw the centiles which we would obtain if they all had the spurt at the same time. To do this, data from children who had been measured repeatedly were used so that the shape of the curve during adolescence in each child and, in particular, the point at which he reached his maximal growth rate (PHV) was seen. The curves were then realigned as in Fig. 4b so that the maximum growth rate during the spurt was at the same age in all children. The age chosen was the average age at PHV for the population. The centiles were calculated after this adjustment had been made, separately for the two sexes.

Charts constructed in this way are known as the "longitudinal" type

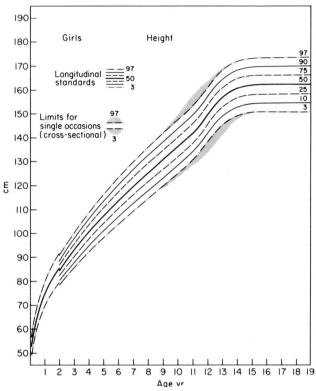

Fig. 20. "Longitudinal" stature centile chart for girls. The shaded areas represent the limits of the corresponding "cross sectional" centiles. Reproduced by kind permission of Professor J. M. Tanner.

(Figs 20 and 21). They show the true shape of the growth curve of a typical adolescent whereas "cross-sectional" type charts (i.e. those in which each individual was measured only once) do not do this. The growth curve of a normal individual will not follow even the longitudinal type centile lines unless he experiences the adolescent growth spurt at the average age. If his spurt is early his curve will rise in relation to the centiles and then, after his spurt, it will revert back to a lower centile, but not necessarily its pre-adolescent one. The curve of a child who experiences the spurt at a later than average age will fall below its original centile until the spurt begins. The most up-to-date charts constructed by Tanner, based on the data of Tanner, et al. (1966) are of the longitudinal type, but the centile lines are surrounded by shading which illustrates the area within which the growth curves of early- and late-maturing children would fall during the adolescent spurt.

Figures 20 to 23 are reproduced on pp. 171, 172 at a larger size, for practical use.

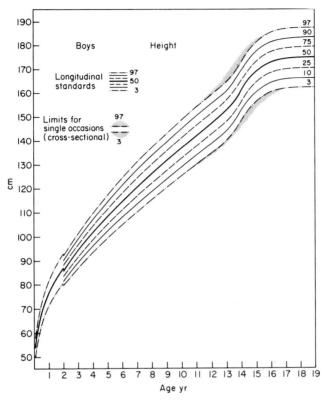

Fig. 21. "Longitudinal" stature centile chart for boys. The shaded areas represent the limits of the corresponding "cross-sectional" centiles. Reproduced from Tanner and Whitehouse (1976) with permission.

Stature Velocity Centiles

Not only do the actual heights of children vary greatly at any given age but the speeds at which they are growing do so as well. Between the 8th and 9th birthdays, for example, some boys will grow 7 cm while others will grow only 4 cm. This variation in growth velocity at each age, like the variation of stature itself, is most conveniently described by centile charts (Figs 22 and 23). The centiles shown on this chart describe the variation in growth velocity in individuals who are measured twice with an interval of one year between measurements. If the time interval between the measurements is less than this, the variation increases. This is due partly to the fact that measurements of growth velocity are relatively less accurate over the shorter periods, because the errors in the two measurements of stature are closer to the actual increase which has occurred (see Chapter 1), and partly to the changes which take

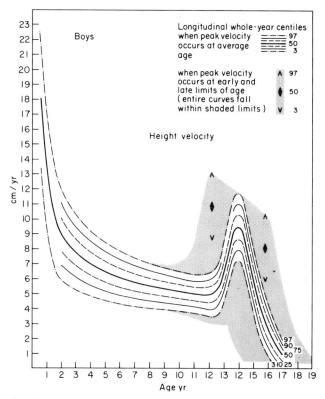

Fig. 22. Centiles of stature velocities in boys who experienced the adolescent spurt at the average age. The shading indicates the area in which the velocities of early- or late-maturing children would fall. Reproduced from Tanner and Whitehouse (1976) with permission.

place in the growth rates of individual children during the course of the year. Some perfectly healthy individuals may not grow at all during a single period of three months, although they may grow fast enough in the remaining nine months to establish a normal velocity over the whole year. Variations in the growth rate occur during the year in most children. They are referred to widely as "seasonal variation" but they probably follow a strictly seasonal pattern in only about 30% of children (Marshall, 1975).

The construction of charts to illustrate growth velocity centiles during the adolescent period is complicated, as with stature centiles, by the occurrence of the adolescent spurt at different ages in different children. In the charts shown in Figs. 22 and 23 the centiles, after the age of 7 in girls and 8 in boys, are those for children who have the spurt at the average age. The surrounding shading covers the area in which early- or late-maturing children would fall. In these children, the shape of the

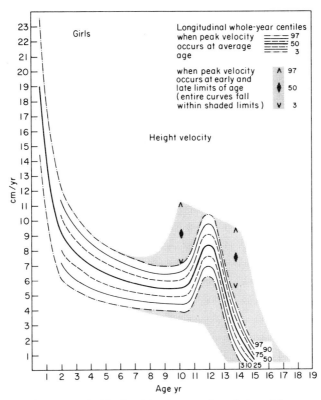

Fig. 23. Centiles of stature velocities in girls who experienced the adolescent spurt at the average age. The shading indicates the area in which the velocities of early- and late-maturing children would fall. Reproduced by kind permission of Professor J. M. Tanner.

adolescent velocity curve is similar to that of the centile lines but is moved to the left in the case of the early maturers or to the right in the case of late maturers. The sloping upper limit of the shading reflects the fact that the maximum growth velocity reached in early-maturing children is usually greater than that attained by late maturers. The velocity curves of an early- and a late-maturing child are shown on a centile chart in Fig. 24.

Repeated measurements of growth velocity in an individual child seldom follow a given centile line unless they are very close to the 50th centile. The chart indicates the range of velocities at which normal children may grow in any one year. A child who grew at, for example, the 10th centile for several years would be falling steadily further below the average stature of his peers. A 10th centile velocity is quite normal for a limited time but it must be compensated by velocities above the

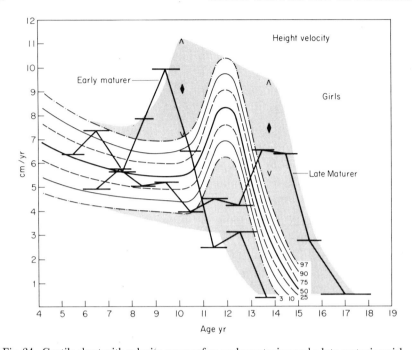

Fig. 24. Centile chart with velocity curves of an early-maturing and a late-maturing girl.

50th centile at other times if satisfactory growth is to be maintained (see Chapter 3).

Weight Centiles

Centiles for weight and weight velocity are shown in Figs 25 to 28 although, as we have mentioned in Chapter 1, a child's weight or weight velocity is a poor guide to his growth. However, a pattern of weight gain which is quite different from that which we would expect in relation to the child's height, may sometimes be of clinical importance.

THE ADOLESCENT GROWTH SPURT

Maximal Growth Velocity

The growth velocity curve of an adolescent rises to a maximum, and then immediately begins to fall again.

The maximum speed (peak height velocity or PHV) reached by different children varies widely. In the Harpenden Growth Study 41 girls were measured every three months by the same skilled observer and a velocity curve was drawn for each subject. Their peak height

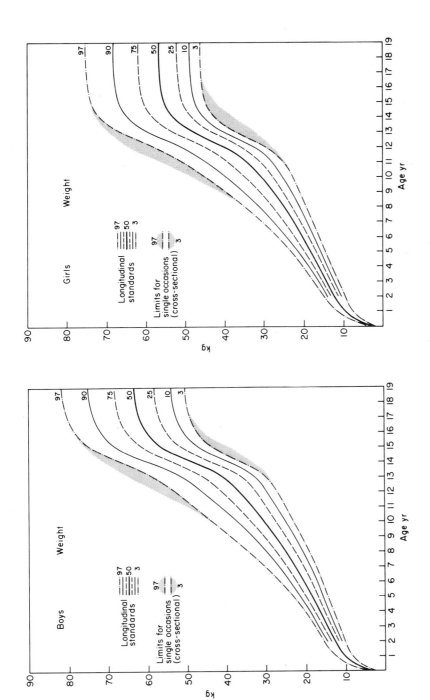

Fig. 25. Weight centiles – boys. Reproduced from Tanner and Whitehouse (1976) with permission.

Fig. 26. Weight centiles – girls. Reproduced by kind permission of Professor J. M. Tanner.

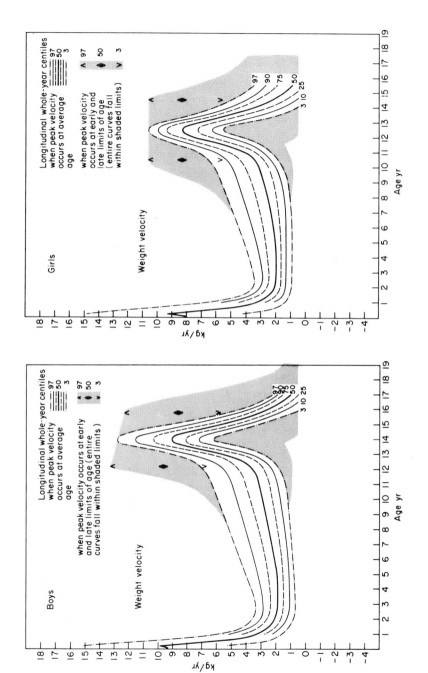

Fig. 27. Weight velocity centiles – boys. Reproduced from Tanner and Whitehouse (1976) with permission.

Fig. 28. Weight velocity centiles – girls. Reproduced by kind permission of Professor J. M. Tanner.

velocities, obtained from these curves, averaged 9·0 cm/yr with a standard deviation of 1·03 cm/yr. Readers who are unfamiliar with the term "standard deviation" should consult an elementary textbook of statistics. In the present context it is sufficient to say that approximately two-thirds of the values in a symmetrically distributed (Gaussian) population are within one standard deviation and only 5% of individuals differ from the mean by more than two standard deviations. For practical purposes therefore, the range of variation is defined by two standard deviations on either side of the mean. Thus girls' peak velocities vary between approximately 7 and 11 cm/yr. However, this maximal velocity is not maintained for any appreciable time and the amount actually gained in the year of fastest growth is less than this. The gain in stature over the whole year centred on the PHV averages 8·4 cm. The mean growth rate immediately before the spurt began was in the region of 5 cm/yr for both these girls, and 49 boys measured in the same study. The average PHV of the boys was 10·3 cm/yr, estimated by drawing a curve through the individual measurements for each one as in the case of the girls. There was a standard deviation of 1·54 cm/yr, which implies an overall range of approximately 7·2 cm/yr to 13·4 cm/yr. The velocity over the whole year, centred on the peak averaged 9·5 cm/yr.

As we have seen above, it is the velocity over the whole year which is important for clinical purposes and which appears as the 50th centile peak velocity on the charts.

Age at Peak Height Velocity

Marshall and Tanner (1969) observed a mean age at peak height velocity of 12·14 ± 0·14 yr (with a standard deviation of 0·88 yr) in a sample of British girls. Thus adolescent girls may reach their maximum growth rates at any time between their 10th and 14th birthdays and few will be outside these limits. For boys, the mean age was 14·06 ± 0·14 yr with an SD of 0·92 yr (Marshall and Tanner, 1970), i.e. most boys reach PHV between their 12th and 16th birthdays.

Sex Difference in Adolescent Growth

Because the adolescent growth spurt occurs on the average about two years earlier in girls than in boys, many girls begin to grow very quickly while the majority of boys of the same age are still growing slowly, at their pre-adolescent rate. These girls become temporarily taller in comparison with boys of their own age. However, as Fig. 29 shows, this effect is relatively slight and is of real importance only to tall girls, who may suddenly find that they are taller than all the boys in their age group, and to small boys who are in the opposite situation, being smaller than all the girls. Fortunately, in most cases, the girl's growth will slow down as that of the boy begins to accelerate and the boys usually become taller in the end. Those children who are nearer to the average size are unlikely to notice the difference at all, particularly as in real life there is a variation of some four years in the age at which the adolescent spurt occurs in both sexes. Many early maturing boys therefore experience accelerated growth before some late maturing girls.

Before puberty there is little difference in stature between girls and boys but boys have a greater adolescent spurt and have two more years of pre-adolescent growth than girls. Thus the boys, even at the beginning of the adolescent spurt, are on the average 10 cm taller than girls at the corresponding stage, who, of course, are younger.

During adolescence, boys' shoulders become much broader, while in

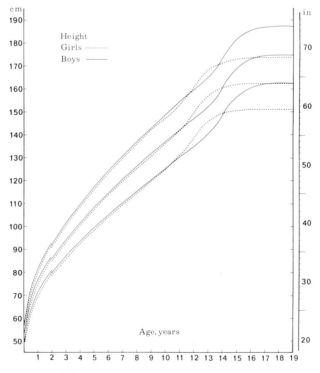

Fig. 29. Growth curves of three girls and three boys in whom the adolescent spurt occurred at the average age for the sex. The discontinuity between the ages of 2 and 3 is caused by the change in measuring technique, from supine length to standing height. Reproduced from Marshall (1970) with permission.

girls there is a greater increase in the width of the hips. In fact, the absolute increase in hip width is the same in the two sexes, but in girls, shoulder widths increase very little and there is less growth of the body as a whole, so that the hips appear wide, in contrast to the boys whose great increase in shoulder width creates the illusion of narrow hips.

Social Implications of Early and Late Maturation

The curves obtained by plotting repeated measurements of four different individuals are shown in Fig. 30. Boy No. 1 was tall in childhood

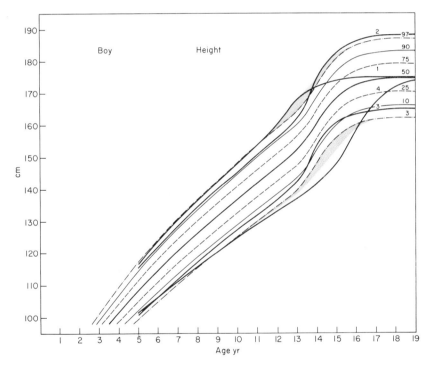

Fig. 30. Centile chart with growth curves of four individuals. Note how the early or late occurrence of the adolescent spurt affected the status of these boys.

but only because he was an early maturer. His tallness in relation to other boys was accentuated between the ages of 12 and 14 by his relatively early adolescent spurt, which brought his growth curve into the shaded part of the chart. However, his growth also began to slow down early and had virtually stopped by his 15th birthday, so that his final stature was not far from the 50th centile. Number 2 was also tall in childhood but was not an early maturer. His growth therefore continued and he became a tall adult.

In contrast, No. 4 was small in childhood because he was a late maturer and his stature fell progressively below the 3rd centile from the age of 11 onwards. Eventually, however, his late adolescent spurt brought his stature to within 3 cm of the 50th centile and not very far from that of No. 1, whilst No. 3, who was not a late maturer, remained small. Thus, two boys with childhood statures near the two extremes of the normal range ended up with very similar adult heights; Nos 1 and 2, on the other hand, were similar in size up to adolescence, but very different as adults.

It is clear from the example of these boys that, when we look at a child's stature on the centile chart we are comparing him only with others of his own age and we cannot make any prediction of his final height. This would involve further consideration of his maturity, as discussed in Chapter 5.

It is worth noting that the range of statures in children of any single age group is much greater than the amount of growth which occurs in any one year. For example, the average increase in stature between the 8th and 9th birthdays is 5 cm but the stature of boys at each of these ages varies by about 20 cm. Therefore a tall (97th centile) 8-year-old is much taller than the average 9-year-old, and is actually taller than some 10% of boys at their 11th birthday, while a small, but perfectly normal child of 9 is no taller than a big 5-year-old. A child's age is thus only a very crude indication of what his stature ought to be.

Variations in the growth of normal children are not only of academic interest. They play an important part in determining the social status of the child within his peer group; while some benefit from their stature others suffer because of it. For example, boy No. 1 in Fig. 30, who was an early maturer, was both taller and stronger than many other boys of his age. These attributes made it easier for him to attain a position of respect and leadership amongst his peers. From the age of 14, however, he began to lose his privileged position because his growth began to slow down, at the same time as many of his peers were entering their adolescent spurts and growing very quickly. Eventually, No. 2, and many other boys, became taller than No. 1.

Number 4, being a late maturer, was not infrequently teased and bullied because he was so small and relatively weak. At the age of 14 to 15 his difficulties became extreme because most of the other boys were developing sexually and becoming rapidly bigger and stronger. None of these things were happening to boy No. 4, who became increasingly handicapped socially. Nevertheless, the final outcome was entirely satisfactory, although his growth in stature and his sexual development were not completed for some time after most of his peers had reached maturity. Number 3, although always rather small, did not suffer the embarrassment of delayed sexual development and physical weakness.

VARIATIONS OF GROWTH IN DIFFERENT PARTS OF THE BODY

The size and velocity curves for body weight and nearly all skeletal dimensions, as well as internal organs and soft tissues, are broadly similar in shape to those for stature. Obviously all parts of the body do not grow at the same absolute rate but most parts grow at a decreasing rate in the first year or so with a few more years of gradual deceleration until the adolescent spurt occurs. However, some dimensions increase more than others during the adolescent spurt and some exhibit the spurt earlier than others.

There are, however, some exceptions to the general growth pattern such as the head, the reproductive organs (see Chapter 4) and the lymphatic tissues (see Chapter 6). Some regions go through the whole growth process more quickly than others. Broadly speaking, the head (which does not exhibit the standard growth pattern) is much more advanced in progress towards its adult size than the trunk while, within the trunk, the shoulder girdle is nearer its adult size at any given time than is the pelvic girdle. This phenomenon has been described as a cranio-caudal "maturity gradient".

This gradient is manifested in the early embryo by the greater development of the cranial than the caudal end. At birth the head is much larger in relation to the rest of the body than it is in later life and constitutes about one-fifth of the child's total length. The legs, at this age, are small. In the limbs, the maturity gradient runs from the distal to the proximal end so that, during childhood, the foot is nearer its adult size at any given age than the leg, which in turn is more advanced in growth than the thigh. A similar situation exists in the upper limb.

Trunk and Limbs

For practical purposes trunk length is usually measured as sitting height (see Chapter 1) and this is subtracted from stature to give the sub-ischial length. At adolescence, the leg length (sub-ischial) reaches its peak growth velocity about six months earlier, on the average, than the trunk. The spurt in sitting height is greater than in the lower limb in normal children and increases the proportion of the total stature that is due to the trunk. As the spurt in stature is due to the acceleration in both trunk length and leg length, peak height velocity is reached when the sum of the velocities of the two segments is maximal. This usually occurs at about the same time as peak velocity in sitting height, but in those children who experience a substantial and earlier acceleration of lower limb length, stature will reach its peak velocity some time after the legs but before the trunk.

Centiles for sitting height are shown in Fig. 31. These are important in clinical work if the lower limbs of a patient are of abnormal length, asymmetrical or deformed and measurements of stature are therefore misleading. When we have to decide, for clinical purposes, whether the limbs are of normal length in relation to the trunk, we usually consider the relationship between sitting height and stature.

The centiles of sitting height in children of given statures (Figs 15 and 16, Chapter 1) give the information we need. It is noteworthy that the sitting height, and hence the length of the legs, may vary by up to 7 cm in children of the same stature, while in young adults of the same stature and sex, leg length may vary up to 12 cm. The upper arm and forearm may both vary by up to 4 cm at a given sitting height.

The foot shows its relatively slight acceleration of growth about six months before the leg, which in turn, accelerates a little earlier than the thigh. The foot usually completes its growth in length before any other part of the limbs or trunk and therefore reaches its adult size before growth in stature is completed. Some adolescents, particularly girls, are concerned because they have large feet when their stature is rapidly increasing. They assume that their feet will continue to grow at comparable rate and become enormous. Fortunately, this seldom happens.

The maturity gradient in the arm is similar to that in the leg and at adolescence the forearm reaches its peak growth velocity about six months before the upper arm, although some individuals show very little spurt at all in the forearm.

The hips and shoulders reach their maximal growth rates at approximately the same time as the trunk.

Head and Face

The cranium exhibits a pattern of post-natal growth quite different from the remainder of the body and approaches its adult size quite early in childhood. Between birth and the age of 18, the circumference of the head increases on the average by about 20 cm. Half this increase has been achieved by the age of eight or nine months and three-quarters by the end of the second year. The remaining growth takes place very

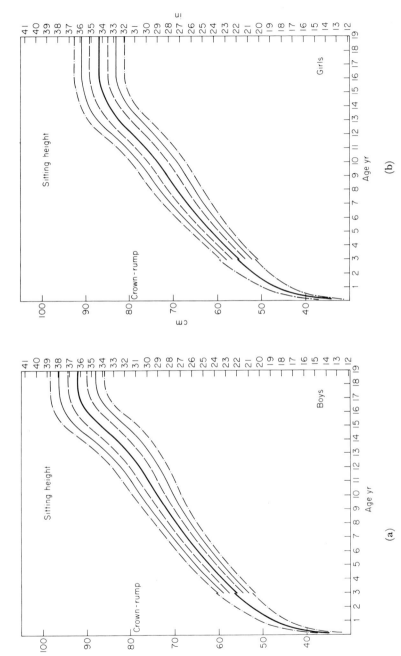

Fig. 31. Centiles for sitting height of (a) boys and (b) girls. Reproduced from Tanner (1973) with permission.

slowly with a detectable, although small, acceleration occurring during adolescence. There is less evidence of a spurt in the length or breadth of the cranium (Fig. 32).

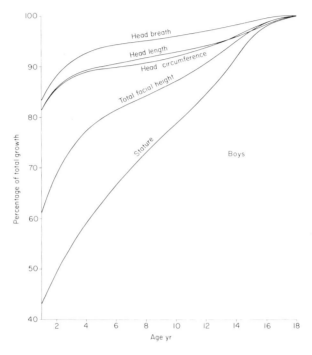

Fig. 32. Growth of various parameters of head and face compared with that of stature in boys. All measurements are expressed as percentages of their adult value. Based on data from Prokopec (1965).

Compression of the head during birth results in overlapping of the bones of the cranial vault and narrowing of the sutures. The resulting distortion makes measurements of head circumference meaningless from the growth point of view. Measurements taken at birth cannot represent the beginning of the postnatal growth process. Much of the increase in head circumference during the neonatal period is due to recovery from moulding, rather than to actual growth of the cranium. The bones usually return to their normal position within a few days of birth and only then is it possible to take measurements which can be compared meaningfully with those taken at later ages.

The normal variation in head circumference is shown in the form of centile charts in Figs 33 and 34. Note that the normal head circumference at the end of the first year varies by 5 cm in girls and 6 cm in

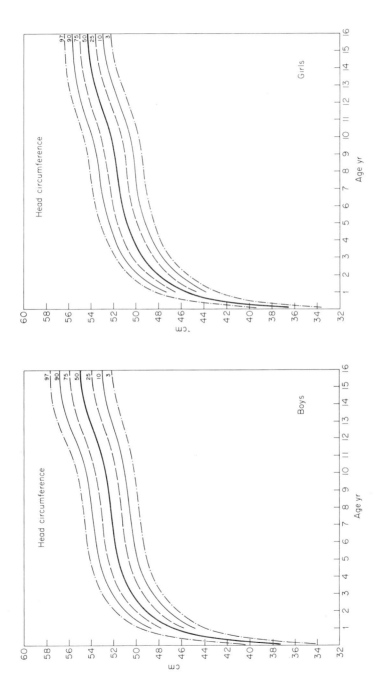

Fig. 33. Centiles of head circumference in boys at different ages. Reproduced from Tanner (1973) with permission.

Fig. 34. Centiles of head circumference in girls at different ages. Reproduced from Tanner (1973) with permission.

boys; the girls' head being on the average 1 cm smaller at this age. With head circumference, as with stature, the rate of growth is often more important than the absolute value. Centiles for head circumference velocity in both sexes are therefore shown in Fig. 35. The velocity of growth in head circumference is expressed in cm/yr and is calculated in the same way as stature velocity.

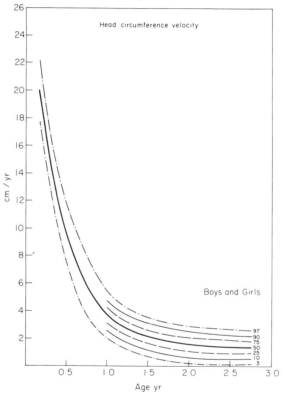

Fig. 35. Velocity (i.e. rate of change in cm/yr) of head circumference in children of both sexes. Reproduced from Tanner (1973) with permission.

At birth, the cranium is much larger than the face and during the first six months or so it grows more quickly than the remainder of the skull, but after this the face begins to grow more quickly.

Some authors have concluded from radiographic studies that the apparent growth of the cranium at adolescence is due almost entirely to increase in the thickness of the bones and the soft tissues of the scalp. However, a more recent radiographic, longitudinal study of head widths from the ages of 9 to 14 showed that, in both sexes, there was very little increase in the thickness of bone. Growth was due mainly to increase in the thickness in the soft tissues and in the width of the cranial cavity. Girls showed more increase in soft tissue while boys showed more growth in the width of the cranial cavity (Singh, *et al.*, 1967).

The forward growth of the forehead at adolescence is due mainly to the development of the brow ridges and frontal sinuses according to Björk (1955) who studied radiographically 243 boys at the age of 12 and again at the age of 20. However, the middle and posterior cranial fossae do enlarge to some extent while the cranial base posterior to the sella turcica increases in length and is lowered.

The height of the cranium increases slowly in later childhood, e.g. by 2 or 3 mm between the ages of 5 and 7 in most children, with a tendency for the growth curve to level out with the passage of time. Nevertheless, a clear adolescent spurt in this dimension has been observed in more than 50% of individuals studied longitudinally.

The inter-orbital distance probably increases slowly throughout childhood with very slight, if any, acceleration at adolescence. The orbits are quite large at birth and nearer to their adult size than any other portion of the face.

The total height of the face increases rapidly during the first two or three years of life and then its growth slows down, like that of the cranium, but there is a definite spurt of growth at adolescence (Fig. 32). This is greater in boys than in girls.

The growth of the whole naso-maxillary complex is directed in a forward and downward direction. During the first year of life the palate and maxilla increase in width by surface apposition but later growth is localized to specific areas. Growth in height and length of the naso-maxillary complex are largely dependent upon alveolar growth in later childhood, but the body of the maxilla also increases in length as a result of sutural growth. Growth of the anterior portions of the palate and maxilla is limited by the closure of the premaxillo-maxillary suture in early infancy. Palatal width is finally fixed by the closure of the sagittal suture round about the fifth year. Surface apposition on the alveolar bone increases the width sufficiently for the development of the molars. Bizygomatic width increases up to the age of about 17.

The mandible grows by apposition at all its surfaces and borders. Its width is increased by symphysial growth but the symphysis closes in the second year. Except for the condylar area, all further growth is due to subperiosteal deposition of bone. Elongation of the condyles pushes the mandible downwards and forwards. While this is happening, resorption takes place on the anterior border of the ramus with deposition along the posterior border, thereby increasing the overall length of the mandible as well as the height of the ramus. The bigonial width also increases as a result of this process because the two halves of the body diverge. The alveolar processes begins to form during the first years of life and its development to full size is dependent upon the presence of the teeth.

The face as a whole grows downwards and forwards in relation to the cranial base but, at birth, the mandible is considerably smaller by comparison with its adult size than is the naso-maxillary complex which, in turn, is smaller than the cranium. Thus, in the head we have a maturity gradient as in other parts of the body. The general forward and downward growth of the whole face is largely dependent upon the mandible growing more quickly than the upper parts. Mandibular growth also continues until a later age.

At puberty most facial dimensions exhibit a spurt. The greatest spurt is in length and height of the mandible where 25% of the total growth in the height of the ramus is completed between the ages of 12 and 20. As a result of this, the jaw becomes considerably longer in relation to the front of the face and projects more prominently. These changes are much more marked in boys than in girls. The adolescent spurt does not, however, complete the growth of the chin as further apposition of bone at the mandibular symphysis usually occurs between 15 and 23 years of age.

The Heart, Lungs and Viscera

The viscera in general show curves of growth similar to those for stature. Radiographic measurements of the transverse diameter of the heart show an adolescent spurt. According to a recent longitudinal study by Simon *et al* (1972) both the diameter of the heart and the width of the lungs reach their maximum rates of growth at approximately the same time as stature reaches its peak velocity. Lung length, however, reaches its peak growth rate about six months later.

The heart diameter usually reaches about 80% of its adult value by the 6th or 7th year while, at this age, lung length and width are only 66% and 62% respectively of their adult values, i.e. there is a much greater increase in the size of the lungs (relative to their size at age 6) during later childhood and adolescence. The lung measurements are unusual in that there is no age at which the average measurements for girls exceeds that of boys, at least in the relatively small number of subjects so far studied.

During childhood the alveolae multiply rapidly so that the area of the air/tissue interface increases from $2 \cdot 8$ m^2 at birth to 32 m^2 at 8 yr and 75 m^2 in the adult. Growth of the lung during the first three years after birth is due mainly to the increase in the number of alveoli, with little change in their size. The alveoli then increase in size although their number also increases up to the age of about eight. After this the number of alveoli does not change but they continue to expand until the growth of the chest wall is completed. After the age of four months, the alveolar outline also increases in complexity and the capillary bed enlarges, thereby further increasing the area available for gaseous interchange, which is more than doubled between the age of 8 and adulthood.

Growth in respiratory function during childhood is essentially a matter of keeping pace with body size, as the basic pattern has already been established within the first few weeks of life. The total lung capacity of the new born is about 150 ml while that of the 16-year-old is about 5,100 ml. This massive increase is reflected in all commonly employed parameters of pulmonary function. Figure 36 shows the

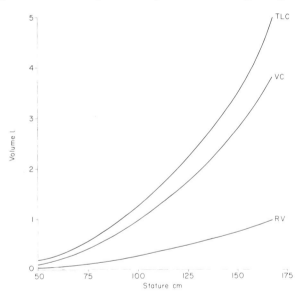

Fig. 36. Typical values of total lung capacity (TLC), vital capacity (VC) and residu a volume (RV) in children of different statures. Data from various sources.

increase in total lung volume, vital capacity and residual volume in relation to height. The figure suggests that the relationship between the total lung capacity and the vital capacity changes very little during growth and, in fact, the residual volume is about 22% of the total lung capacity throughout childhood.

The liver, kidneys, pancreas and the non-lymphatic portion of the spleen probably undergo some spurt in growth at adolescence but the evidence for this is very limited.

3

Detection of Abnormal Growth

INTRODUCTION

The recognition of abnormal growth, as distinct from its differential diagnosis, involves only two basic steps.

i) Measure the child's stature accurately and plot the result against his age on a centile chart (see Chapter 2).

ii) Repeat this procedure as often as is necessary and (using a velocity centile chart), ascertain whether or not the patient's rate of growth is normal.

Stature, or supine length in the child who is too young to stand, is the only measurement which gives an adequate basis for deciding whether a child's overall growth is normal or abnormal. Weight is not a reliable measure for this purpose because the weight of an abnormally short, but obese, child may be within normal limits for his age. Also a child who is growing very little may gain a lot of weight whilst one who is growing quite normally may gain very little weight or even lose some (see Chapter 1).

It should be noted that the years on the "age" axes of the centile charts (Figs 20 to 23) are divided into ten parts and not 12 months. It is standard practice in growth work to divide the year into ten parts and express dates as decimals. This greatly simplifies the calculation of ages and of the time intervals between repeated measurements (see Chapter

54

1). Table I shows the decimal equivalent of each calendar date within the year and this decimal can be preceded by the year itself. For example, 6th January 1963 is 63·014 and 8th July 1975 is 75·515. Thus the age on 8th July 1975 of a child who was born on 6th January 1963 is 75·515 minus 63·014 = 12·501 (or 12·50, taking it to the nearest 3·65 days). It is a worthwhile practice to record the decimal of each child's birthday on his case notes and to enter the decimal equivalent of each day's date in one's diary.

There is no absolute rule about the centile below which a child's stature must fall before he should be regarded as abnormally short. This judgement must be made in each individual case after other factors, discussed below, have been taken into account.

INFLUENCE OF PARENTAL HEIGHT

A child with a stature above the third centile might be regarded as abnormally short if he had very tall parents but the son or daughter of 3rd centile parents might be below this centile, and yet still be normal. Charts are now available (Tanner, et al., 1970) which take parental stature into account and give centiles for the statures of children of given age and "mid-parent height". The mid-parent height is the arithmetic mean of the statures of the two parents. These charts (Figs 37 and 38) are available only for the age range of 2 to 9 years. At any other age we must rely on common sense.

In order to use the charts, look first at the left-hand side, identify the vertical line corresponding to the child's age and the curved line representing his stature. From the point of intersection of these lines, a ruler is placed parallel to the horizontal lines, with its far end in the right side of the chart. The point where this ruler crosses the vertical line corresponding to the average height of the two parents (mid-parent height) is marked. By reference to the diagonal centile lines, the centile position of this point is read and represents the status of the child when the height of his parents have been taken into account. Thus a child at, for example, the 10th centile on this chart has a stature greater than that of 10% of children whose parents are of the same average height as his own.

A child who is measured repeatedly and remains in the same centile channel on the standard centile chart will also remain in the same channel on the chart relating centiles to parental height. If he rises through the centiles on the height for age chart, his position on the new chart will also rise and vice versa.

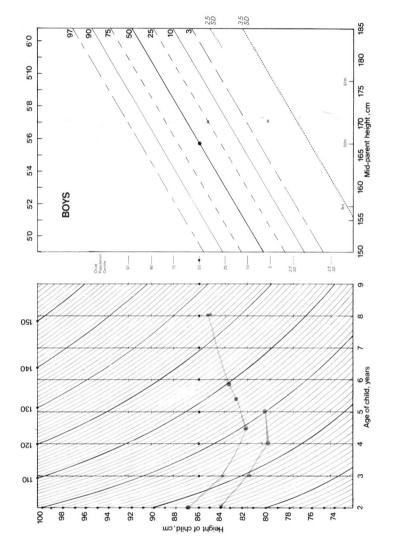

Fig. 37. Variation in boys' heights at ages 2 to 9 years, allowing for height of parents. Reproduced from Tanner *et al.* (1970) with permission.

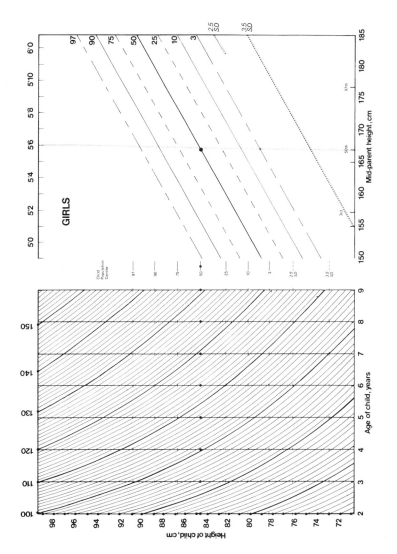

Fig. 38. Variation in girls' heights at ages 2 to 9 years, allowing for height of parents. Reproduced from Tanner *et al.* (1970) with permission.

THE IMPORTANCE OF REPEATED MEASUREMENTS

Even a child who is well within the centiles for stature may not be growing normally. If the growth of a tall child slows down, or even stops, it may be a long time before this set-back becomes apparent on the centile chart as abnormally short stature. To recognize this kind of situation, which is usually indicative of some major disorder, we must measure the child more than once. Figure 39 shows the growth curve of

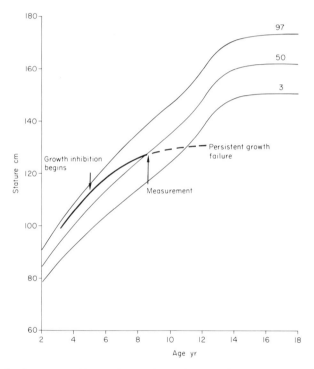

Fig. 39. Centiles for stature with superimposed growth curve of a tall girl who suffered growth inhibition from the age of five years and whose growth had virtually stopped by the age of 8·5. Note that a single measurement of stature at age 8·5 would not have revealed any abnormality in her growth.

a girl who was at the 90th centile up to the age of 5, when her growth began to slow down. By the time she was 8½ years old her growth had virtually stopped but a single measurement at that time would have shown her stature to be at the 50th centile i.e. "average" and therefore "normal". The solid part of the growth curve indicates what actually happened before the measurement was taken. The fact that her growth was grossly abnormal would have been revealed if a second measurement had been taken later. This would have shown that her growth was following a path indicated by the interrupted line and that her growth rate was abnormally low.

STATURE VELOCITY AS AN INDICATOR OF ABNORMAL GROWTH

It is clear from the above example that an essential part of our assessment of a child's growth is to discover whether or not he is growing at a normal speed. It is particularly important that we should recognize abnormally slow growth, even if the child's present stature is within normal limits, because it may indicate an underlying disorder requiring treatment. The growth velocity, preferably over a whole year, must be calculated from repeated measurements and plotted on a velocity chart (see Chapter 2).

If a child's growth rate for the whole year is below the 50th centile, even if it is well above the 3rd centile, he is losing ground in relation to the average child of his own age. Thus, if he is already small, he is becoming relatively smaller and he must grow at a rate above the 50th centile in some future year if he is to maintain his status in the population. In the case of a tall child a rate below the 50th centile will bring his stature nearer to the average. Only those whose growth rates are near the 50th centile should maintain the same status on the velocity centile chart.

Figure 40 shows the growth in stature which would occur in three

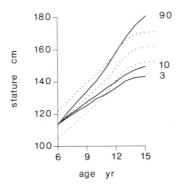

Fig. 40. Growth in stature of three hypothetical girls whose growth remained consistently on the 3rd, 10th and 90th centiles for velocity from the age of six onwards. The dotted lines show the 3rd, 10th and 97th centiles for stature. Reproduced from Marshall (1974b) with permission of W. B. Saunders and Co. Ltd.

hypothetical girls who were on the 50th centile for stature on their 6th
birthdays but grew consistently at the 3rd, 10th and 90th centiles for
velocity. Although the growth rate of each of these children is within
normal limits in any one year, in total they result in abnormal growth.
As we saw in Chapter 2, it is difficult to reach a firm conclusion about a
child's growth rate if we have observed him for less than a year. This is
due partly to the fact that the measurement of growth velocity is less
accurate over a short interval of time and partly to the periodic variation in growth rate which occurs in many normal children. The only
way to eliminate these variations when assessing the growth of an individual child is to calculate his growth velocity over a period which is
close to a whole year. The standard velocity centile charts are based on
parts of measurements, taken at intervals of almost exactly a year, in
individual children. A velocity which is abnormally low in relation to
these charts, but has been measured over a period of much less than a
year, does not necessarily indicate abnormal growth. It does mean that
the child should be observed for a longer period, and, if the overall
clinical picture warrants it, some preliminary investigations might be
carried out.

4

Puberty

INTRODUCTION

Puberty is a combination of anatomical and physiological changes including the maturation of the gonads, acceleration of somatic growth (the adolescent spurt), the development of the secondary sex characters and other physiological changes. These events take place at ages which vary widely between different individuals. The time which elapses from their onset to their completion and the sequence in which they occur are also variable.

DEVELOPMENT OF REPRODUCTIVE ORGANS AND SECONDARY SEX CHARACTERS IN GIRLS

Vagina and Uterus

The earliest clinical indication that a girl is approaching puberty is an increase in the number of superficial cells in her vaginal smear. This may be found before there are any other signs of sexual development or before the mucosa of the vulva shows any macroscopic sign of stimulation by oestrogen. At about the same time the vagina begins to lengthen and it continues to do so until menarche, the beginning of the first menstrual period, or a little later. The endometrium develops over approximately the same period of time as the secondary sex characters. Any growth that occurs in the body of the uterus before puberty is mainly confined to the myometrium.

Apocrine Glands

The apocrine glands in the axilla and vulva begin to function at puberty. There is no exact information about the ages at which this may occur in different girls but increasing apocrine secretion is apparently related to the development of the pubic and axillary hair. The sebaceous and merocrine sweat glands become more active at about the same time.

Breasts

For descriptive purposes the changes which take place in the breasts during adolescence may be divided into five stages based on their superficial appearance, see Fig. 41 (Tanner, 1962).

> Stage 1 (B1): This is the infantile stage which persists from the time the effect of maternal oestrogen on the breasts disappears, shortly after birth, until the changes of puberty begin.
> Stage 2 (B2): The bud stage. The breasts and papilla are elevated as a small mound and there is an increase in the diameter of the areola. This stage represents the first indication of pubertal change in the breast.
> Stage 3 (B3): The breasts and areola are further enlarged to create an appearance similar to that of a small adult breast, with a continuous rounded contour.
> Stage 4 (B4): The areola and papilla enlarge further to form a secondary mound projecting above the contour of the remainder of the breast.
> Stage 5 (B5): The typical adult breast with smooth rounded contour. The secondary mound present in stage 4 has disappeared.

The time at which a girl's breasts first attain the appearance described above as a "stage" is usually indicated by the corresponding abbreviation B2, B3 etc.

Some girl's breasts do not develop beyond the appearance described in stage 4 until the first pregnancy, and never attain stage 5. Alternatively, there are a few girls who apparently pass directly from stage 3 to stage 5 without exhibiting the characteristics of stage 4, or having done so for less than three months (Marshall and Tanner, 1969). These authors also noted a return to stage 4 in three out of 70 girls who had previously been described as stage 5.

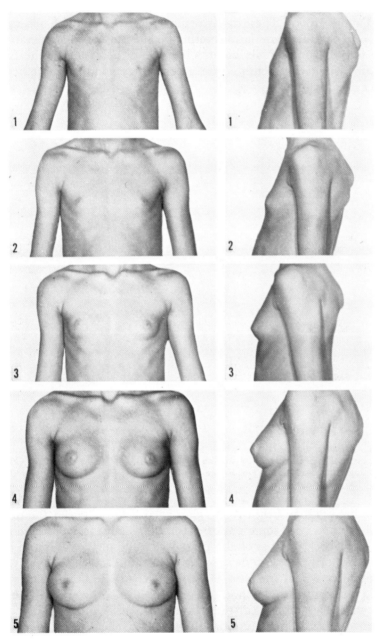

Fig. 41. Stages of breast development. Reproduced from Tanner (1962) with permission.

Figure 42 shows the range of ages at which each stage of breast development is reached in 95% of British girls, as estimated by Marshall and Tanner (1969). These data are in good agreement with observations from other similar populations although the mean age of menarche for this sample was about six months later than the mean for the London girls. Breast development may have been correspondingly late but there is no evidence about this.

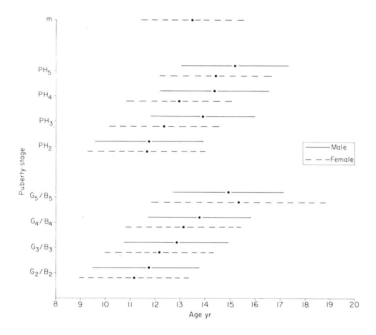

Fig. 42. Variation in age within which 95% of children reach various stages of sexual development. The central point in each horizontal line represents the mean. G2, G3 etc. = genital stages in boys; B2, B3, etc. = breast stages in girls; PH2, PH3, etc. = pubic hair stages; M = menarche.

The breasts may begin to develop at any age between the 9th and 13th birthdays with some 5% of normal girls outside even these limits. In a typical school class of about 30 9-year-old girls, we should expect to find two or three with developing breasts and, as the year advances, this number would increase to about ten. At the other extreme, we should not be surprised to find two or three girls without breast development in a class of 13-year-olds. Some girls have fully mature breasts before their 12th birthdays but others do not reach breast stage 5 until they are 19 or even older.

Pubic Hair

The development of pubic hair like that of the breasts may be described in five stages (Fig. 43).

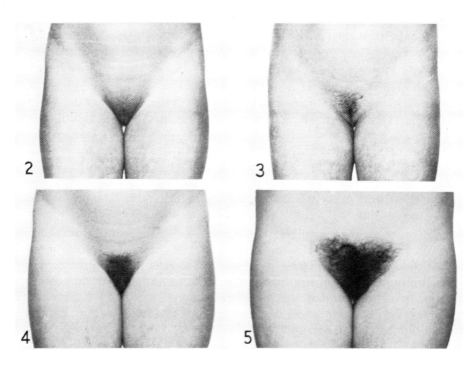

Fig. 43. Stages of pubic hair growth (these are the same for both sexes). Stage 1, in which there is no growth of hair, is not illustrated. Reproduced from Tanner (1975) with permission.

Stage 1 (PH1): The infantile stage, in which there is no true pubic hair growth although there may be a downy vellus similar to that on the abdominal wall.

Stage 2 (PH2): Sparse growth of slightly pigmented hairs on either the labia or the mons pubis.

Stage 3 (PH3): The hair is darker and coarser and spreads sparsely over, and on either side of, the mid line of the mons pubis.

Stage 4 (PH4): The hair is adult in character but covers a smaller area than in most adults and has not spread to the medial surface of the thighs.

Stage 5 (PH5): Hair distributed as an inverse triangle and spreading to the medial surfaces of the thighs. It does not spread to the linea alba or elsewhere above the base of the triangle.

For practical purposes stage 5 may be regarded as the completion of pubic hair growth at puberty, although in about 10% of women, hair later spreads upwards onto the abdominal wall.

The first appearance of each of the stages is usually indicated by the abbreviations, PH2, PH3, etc. 95% of West European girls reach the various stages of pubic hair growth within the range of ages shown in Fig. 42. Pubic hair growth may begin in girls at any age from about 8·5 onwards and the adult distribution of hair (PH5) is usually attained between the ages of 12 and 17.

Although it is important to know at what age girls may reach (or enter) a given stage of breast or pubic hair development, as shown in Fig. 42, this information is of limited value in the clinical situation where we are seeing a girl for the first time and want to know if her sexual development is normal for her age. In this case we know what stage the patient is in but we do not know when she reached that stage. For example, if her breasts are in stage 2 all we know is that she reached B2 at some time in the past and has not yet reached B3. The breast bud may have begun to develop a few days ago, or a year ago.

In order to overcome this difficulty, and create standards which would be more useful in a clinical setting, the charts shown in Fig. 44 have been prepared. These illustrate centiles for the ages at which children may be seen in different stages. In using them we do not say "the age of this patient is x therefore in what stage should she be?" We say, for example, "she is in breast stage 3. Is her age within normal limits for a girl in this stage?"

By projecting from her age, on the x-axis, to the bar representing breast stage 3, we can see at which centile she lies. Let us say that she is exactly 13·0 years old and therefore at the 25th centile. This means that 25% of girls in breast stage 3 are older than our patient. Therefore we should have no reason to regard her as abnormal. Had she been 15 years old we should have found that her age was beyond the 3rd centile and would have concluded that she was unusually old for a girl in breast stage 3. On the other hand, if she had been only 9 years old, i.e. just beyond the 97th centile, we would have concluded that she was unusually young for a girl in this stage.

It is important to recognize the distinction between the point in time denoted by, for example, B2 at which the breasts first acquire the appearance defined as stage 2, and the period following this when the appearance has not changed sufficiently to meet the criteria for stage 3. During this time, which may be a year or more, we describe the breasts as "in stage 2".

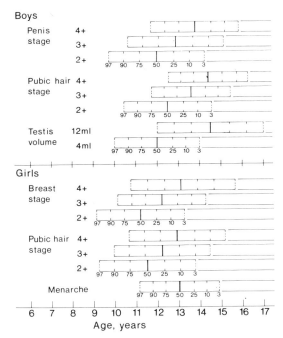

Fig. 44. Centiles for age in given stages of sexual development.

Menarche

The average age at menarche in the southern part of the United Kingdom is 13·0 yr with a standard deviation of approximately one year, thus 95% of the population experience their first menses between their 11th and 15th birthdays. However, the mean age at menarche varies greatly between different populations and, in many countries, there are wide differences between social groups.

Table IV shows the mean age at menarche in various populations. All these values are estimated by the so-called "status quo" method. This is the only satisfactory technique for estimating the age of menarche in populations and is also one of the easiest. All that it requires is to ask each subject how old she is and whether or not she has begun to menstruate. A table is constructed giving the percentage of "yes" and "no" answers at each age. The mean and standard deviation of the age at menarche in the population can be estimated from this data by relatively simple statistical methods, involving probit or logit transformation, which are beyond the scope of this text. The sample of girls questioned must, of course, be sufficiently large and representative of

TABLE IV

Age at menarche in various populations

Country	Year	Mean age
Australia (Sydney)	1970	13.0
Canada (Montreal)	1969	13.1
Chile (Santiago)	1970	12.6
Cuba (Havana)	1973	12.8
(rural)	1973	13.3
Egypt (Nubians)	1966	15.2
England (London)	1966	13.0
Finland	1969	13.2
India (Lucknow)	1967	14.5
Iraq (Baghdad – well off)	1969	13.6
(Baghdad – poorly off)	1969	14.0
Italy (rural)	1969	12.5
Japan	1966–7	12.9
New Guinea (Bundi – highlands)	1967	18.0
(Kaipit – lowlands)	1967	15.6
New Zealand (Maori)	1969	12.7
(non-Maori)	1969	13.0
Norway (Oslo)	1970	13.2
Poland (rural)	1967	14.0
Senegal (Dakar)	1970	14.6
U.S.A. (European origin)	1968	12.5
(African origin)	1968	12.8
U.S.S.R. (Moscow)	1970	13.0

the population. This method does not tell us the actual age at menarche in any individual but gives us the best estimate for the population as a whole.

Other methods, for example, where each subject is asked at what age she began to menstruate, are unreliable. The recollected age is frequently inaccurate and some girls may give deliberately false answers. Also, the result will be biased if the sample includes girls who had not begun to menstruate at the time of the survey. They would be excluded from the calculation because they have no information to contribute. However, their actual age at menarche must be later than their age at the time of the survey and, were it known, would increase the value of the mean. The result obtained when these girls are omitted will therefore be lower than the true value. Wilson and Sutherland (1949) showed that the difference in recalled menarcheal age in two samples of girls was due to the inclusion of more premenarcheal girls in the sample having the lower mean.

A longitudinal study, in which the same subjects are seen repeatedly and are asked on each occasion if they have begun to menstruate, can give reliable information. If the interval between visits is short, the exact date of menarche for each individual can be determined but, for financial and administrative reasons, it is not usually possible to apply this method to sufficiently large or representative samples to provide reliable estimates of the mean for the population.

Age at Menarche in Different Populations. In many countries, menarche occurs at different ages in different socio-economic groups. For example, in the Netherlands, de Wijn (1966) found a mean age of 13·8 yr for girls with poor parents as compared with 13·5 for the parents on the higher social classes. In the United Kingdom there is a variation of about six months between various parts of the country but, in London, after allowance has been made for the number of children in the family, no further effect of social class *per se* is apparent.

Girls of different races experience menarche at different mean ages but it is difficult to determine how much of this diversity is due to race itself and how much to dissimilarity in nutrition, culture and climate. However, some of the variation is apparently due to race as indicated by the fact that Chinese girls living in poverty in Hong Kong, menstruate as early as Europeans in much better economic circumstances (Lee *et al.*, 1963), while the well-off Chinese do so earlier than Europeans. Girls in south-eastern Europe usually reach menarche earlier than West Europeans of similar economic status. Africans of the more privileged groups are similar in this respect to Europeans but those living in poorer conditions (e.g. South African Bantu) have much later mean ages at menarche. The Bundi of New Guinea are very late and constitute the only known group in which menarche nowadays is as late as it was in the rural populations of Europe a hundred years ago.

Roberts (1969) studied the effects of climate on the age at menarche in a number of different racial groups including Europeans, East Asians, Indians and Africans. In any one race, menarche tended to be earlier amongst girls living in higher mean ambient temperatures but, when allowance was made for this, there was still a significant difference between the means for the various racial groups. Menarche is usually later at higher rather than lower altitudes and usually later in rural than in urban communities. Girls in large families tend to experience menarche later than those with fewer brothers and sisters but, within a family, there is a tendency for girls who are born later to reach menarche earlier, by about 0·1 yr for every older sibling (Roberts and Dann, 1967).

During the past century the age at menarche in Europe, North America and some other parts of the world has become progressively earlier at an apparent rate of three or four months for each decade (Fig. 45). Some of the earlier estimates are, of course, not very reliable, but there is such consistency in the apparent trend in different countries

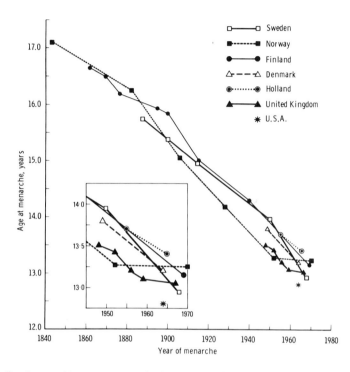

Fig. 45. Secular trend in age at menarche from 1840–1970. Reproduced from Tanner (1975) by kind permission of the author and W. B. Saunders Co. Ltd.

that there is little doubt of its reality. In many countries this trend is apparently continuing but there is evidence that it may be stopping in London and Oslo (Tanner, 1973b; Bruntland and Walløe, 1973).

VARIATION IN THE RATE OF PROGRESS THROUGH SEXUAL DEVELOPMENT IN GIRLS

Children vary greatly not only in the ages at which their secondary sex characters begin to develop but also in the time which they take to pass through the whole sequence of changes which lead to sexual maturity. If we know the age at which a girl attained a given stage of breast development, we still do not know when she will reach the following one. Table V gives the 5th, 50th and 97th centiles of the length of

TABLE V
Lengths of time for which children may remain in various
stages of sexual development
(Based on data from Marshall and Tanner, 1969 and 1970.)

	Years		
	3rd Centile	50th Centile	97th Centile
Girls			
B2	0·2	0·9	1·0
B3	0·1	0·9	2·2
B4	0·1	2·0	6·8
B2 – B5	1·5	4·0	9·0
PH2	0·2	0·6	1·3
PH3	0·2	0·5	0·9
PH4	0·6	1·3	2·4
PH2 – PH5	1·4	2·5	3·1
Boys			
G2	0·4	1·1	2·2
G3	0·2	0·8	1·6
G4	0·4	1·0	1·9
G2 – G5	1·9	3·1	4·7
PH2	0·1	0·4	0·9
PH3	0·3	0·4	0·5
PH4	0·2	0·7	1·5
PH2 – PH5	0·8	1·6	2·7

time for which a girl may remain in a given stage of breast or pubic hair development. For example, the duration of stage 2 is the interval between the attainment of B2 and the attainment of B3 and, on the average, is 0·9 yr. However, some 5% of girls remain in stage 2 for only 0·2 yr or less, while, at the other extreme, there are some who remain in this stage for well over a year. The whole process of breast development, from the first appearance of stage 2 to the attainment of stage 5 takes four years on the average, but this time is very variable, as the table shows. The time which girls may spend in each of the pubic hair stages varies in much the same way.

The average time interval between the first indication of breast development and the first menstrual period is about two and a half years. Menarche rarely occurs less than a year after the breasts have begun to develop but may not do so for over five. The length of this interval does not seem to be related to the age at which breast development begins. Thus, a girl's age when her breasts begin to develop gives us very little information about when we may expect her to experience menarche. Also, a girl whose breasts begin to develop earlier than those of her friend, may experience menarche after her.

INTERRELATIONSHIPS OF THE CHANGES OF PUBERTY IN GIRLS

The breasts and pubic hair do not usually begin to develop simultaneously and they seldom progress at the same rate toward the adult state. Marshall and Tanner (1969) examined 88 normal girls within three months after their pubic hair had begun to develop. 16% had no breast development and 49% were already in breast stage 2. Most of the remainder were in stage 3, but 8% of the total number of girls were in breast stage 4 when pubic hair began to appear. Thus a girl whose breasts are in stage 4, but who has no pubic hair, is not necessarily abnormal. On the other hand, pubic hair may appear before the breasts begin to develop. Of 89 girls who were examined within 3 months after their breasts began to develop (B2), 39% already had pubic hair and two of these were in PH4. Thus the widely-held view that breast development always precedes pubic hair growth in normal girls is quite wrong. Axillary hair also is sometimes present before there is any breast development but it usually does not appear until the breasts are in stage 3 or 4.

Menarche usually occurs when the breasts are in stage 4 but some 25% of girls experience their first menses while they are in breast stage 3, and another 10% approximately, do not menstruate until after their breasts have reached stage 5. This last group of girls, with mature breasts and no periods, sometimes presents a clinical problem. If they are over 15 years old, so that their menarche is also late in terms of chronological age, we have to question whether they are likely to menstruate at all, or whether we should regard them as cases of primary amenorrhoea. The problem would be simplified if we could say that menarche should occur within a certain period of time after B5 has been reached, but this information is not available. The most useful guide in these circumstances is the bone age. If the bone age (as estimated by the TW2 method which is discussed in Chapter 5) is more than 14·5 "years" there is a high probability of primary amenorrhoea, but if the bone age is less than this there is still room for hope that menarche will occur spontaneously. The relationship of bone age to other aspects of sexual development is discussed more fully below.

In most girls the adolescent growth spurt is coincident with the early stages of breast development and about 40% reach their maximum rates of growth in height (PHV) (see Chapter 2) before their breasts have developed beyond stage 2. Therefore we cannot assume that a girl with early breast development is at the beginning of her growth spurt. She may be already approaching PHV or her growth may even have begun to slow down. A further 50% of girls, approximately, reach PHV while their breasts are in stage 3 and only 10% do not do so until their breasts are in stage 4. In this respect, girls differ markedly from boys, who do not usually reach PHV before their genitalia are well developed, i.e. stage 4 (see below).

Menarche seldom, if ever, occurs before the peak of height spurt has been reached. For practical purposes, if we know that a girl has begun to menstruate, we can assume that her growth is slowing down and will continue to do so until it finally stops. The average gain in stature after menarche is approximately 7·3 cm and varies in different girls between about 3 and 11 cm (Singleton *et al.*, 1975).

THE REPRODUCTIVE ORGANS AND SECONDARY SEX CHARACTERS IN BOYS

Testes

The volume of the testes may be measured with the "Prader Orchidometer" (Fig. 46). This is a series of plastic or wooden models of a shape similar to that of the testes and mounted on a length of cord in order of increasing size. The volume in ml of each model is marked on it. The model nearest in size to the testis is identified by palpating the testis with one hand and the models with the other. The volume of this model is read. In pre-adolescent boys, this volume is usually 1, 2 or 3 ml and a volume greater than this usually indicates that puberty is beginning. Nearly all the growth of the testes occurs during puberty. The variation in the size of the testes in boys of different ages is shown in Fig. 47.

There are no Leydig cells in the interstitial tissue of the testes during childhood but, at puberty, increasing quantities of androgen, and possibly oestrogen are produced by Leydig cells, differentiated from the interstitial mesenchyme.

The seminiferous tubules of the infant are cord-like in structure with a diameter of between 50 and 80 μm. They grow slowly and, although the number of spermatogonia increases gradually, the Sertoli cells remain undifferentiated. The first signs of a lumen usually appear in the tubules round about the age of 6 but this lumen does not become distinct until puberty. The division of the basal spermatogonia is the first stage in the sequence of changes in the germinal epithelium which leads

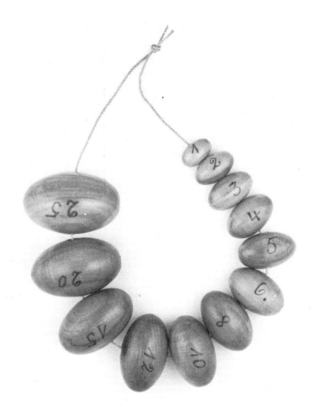

Fig. 46. The Prader Orchidometer.

gradually to spermatogenesis. When the testes are mature, about two-thirds of the lining of the tubules consists of germinal epithelium while the remainder is made up of Sertoli cells.

The epididymis, seminal vesicles and prostate remain infantile in size until the time of puberty when they grow rapidly as they develop functionally.

Penis and Scrotum

The development of the male genitalia, like that of the breasts in girls, may be described as passing through five stages as shown in Fig. 48 (Tanner, 1962).

Pubic Hair

The five stages of pubic hair development in boys are based on the same criteria as are used for girls (Fig. 43) with allowance for the basic anatomical differences. In most men, the pubic hair spreads beyond the triangular pattern which we call stage 5 and some authors describe hair that has spread higher on to the abdominal wall as "stage 6". However, it is convenient to regard stage 5 as the final stage of pubertal development as the hair seldom reaches its fully adult distribution before the age of 20. The variation in the age at which boys reach the various stages of pubic hair growth is shown in Fig. 42.

Axillary and Facial Hair

Axillary hair usually appears a year or two after pubic hair growth has begun and seldom before the development of the genitalia is well advanced. However, this relationship is very variable and axillary hair sometimes appears before there is any growth of hair on the pubis. Facial hair of the adult type usually makes its first appearance at the corner of the upper lip when the genitalia are quite well developed and at about the same time as axillary hair begins to grow. The moustache is gradually completed and, about the same time, hair appears on the upper part of the cheek and just below the lower lip, in the midline. The chin is usually the last site on which hair appears. Hair seldom grows on the chin before the development of the genitalia has been completed.

The Breast

The areola of the male breast increases in diameter at puberty. This change is permanent and is frequently accompanied by temporary enlargement of the underlying breast tissue. This is usually slight, although it may cause some discomfort, and seldom persists for more than a year or so. Occasionally, however, it may persist or even increase and on those rare occasions when the enlargement is sufficient to cause psychological or social problems, surgical treatment may be required.

VARIATION IN RATE OF PROGRESS THROUGH SEXUAL DEVELOPMENT IN BOYS

The duration of a given stage of genital or pubic development in a boy is defined as the difference between the age at which he reached that stage and the age at which he reached the following one. For example, the duration of genital stage 2 is the age (or date) at which he attained stage G3 minus the age (or date) at which he attained G2. The 2·5, 50 and 97·5 centiles for the duration of the genital and pubic hair stages are shown in Table V. Some boys remain for up to $2\frac{1}{2}$ yr in genital stage 2 while others may complete the whole process of their genital development (from G2 to G5) in a shorter time than this. On the other hand, the time which elapses between G2 and G5 may be up to five years and occasionally longer in some subjects. There is no clear relationship between the age at which genital development begins (G2) and the time which elapses before the changes are completed, (G5). Therefore, as in the case of the girls, the fact that we know when a boy began his sexual development does not imply that we know when he will reach maturity. Of two boys, the first to reach genitalia stage 2 need not be the first to reach maturity.

INTERRELATIONSHIPS OF THE CHANGES OF PUBERTY IN BOYS

At any given time the genitalia and pubic hair are not necessarily at the same stage of development. Very few boys experience growth of the pubic hair before their genitalia have begun to develop and some perfectly normal boys are still without pubic hair by the time their genitalia have reached stage 4.

The relationship of the adolescent growth spurt to genital development is also variable. Boys rarely, if ever, reach peak height velocity before their genitalia are in stage 3 and the great majority do so when they are in genital stage 4, although some 20% of boys do not attain their maximal rates of growth until their genitalia are fully mature (stage 5). Thus, in boys, the peak of the adolescent growth spurt is a late event in the sequence of changes at puberty. This contrasts with the situation in girls who quite frequently reach PHV while they are in breast stage 2.

Van Wieringen *et al.* (1968) has shown that the size of the testes varies greatly amongst boys in any given stage of development of the penis and scrotum. This variation was 3 to 9 ml in stage 2, 7 to 16 ml in stage 3, 12 to 24 ml in stage 4 and 16 to 27 ml in adults. Twenty per cent of the population were estimated to be either above or below these limits.

SEX DIFFERENCE IN AGE AT PUBERTY

We have already noted that the adolescent spurt occurs, on the average, about two years earlier in girls than in boys, but this does not necessarily imply that the development of the secondary sex characters is earlier in girls by the same amount. The evidence that is now available suggests that boys' genitalia begin to develop, on the average, only a few months later than the girls' breasts and may reach maturity at about the same age as the girls breasts reach stage 5. Of course the variation within each sex is so great that an early maturing boy may begin to develop four years or so before a late maturing girl and vice versa.

However, from the social point of view, the apparent difference between boys and girls in the age at puberty is perhaps more important than any strict biological difference. Puberty is obvious to untrained observers at an earlier age in girls than in boys, because girls' earlier adolescent growth spurt makes them taller and the development of their breasts is visible even when they are fully clothed. The genital development, which is occurring in boys at the same time, is not visible in most social situations and those changes which can be easily recognized, such as the breaking of the voice and the appearance of the facial hair, do not occur until much later. Thus a typical girl becomes an obvious adolescent, from the social point of view, a year or two before the corresponding boy shows any evidence of approaching manhood.

RELATIONSHIP OF SKELETAL AND SEXUAL MATURATION

The methods used to estimate the maturity of a child's skeleton are discussed in Chapter 6. This aspect of maturity may be expressed as a "bone age" which, taken in conjunction with the child's stature, may be used to predict his or her adult stature with an accuracy which, although not great, is sufficient for many clinical purposes.

It is often assumed that skeletal age may also be used to predict when the changes of puberty will begin. A child with an advanced skeletal age is expected to reach puberty earlier than one whose skeletal age is much less than his chronological age. This assumption is partly justified where the advancement is extreme, as in precocious puberty and, probably, also in extreme delay. However, it does not apply within the normal range of variation. Marshall (1974a) determined the skeletal ages of some 70 girls and 100 boys when they attained various stages of sexual development. When girls reached breast stage 2 (B2) their skeletal ages varied between 8 and 14 "years" while at breast stage 5 (B5) they varied between 12 and 16. Thus the variation in skeletal age was very similar to that in chronological age and clearly indicates that there is no simple relationship between the ossification of the skeleton and the development of the breasts. Menarche, however, is apparently related in some way to skeletal maturation as approximately 85% of the girls had bone ages of between 13 and 14 "years" when they experienced their first menses.

Most girls reached 95% of their mature height at bone ages close to 13 "years", but at the peak of the adolescent growth spurt (PHV) the bone age varied between 10 "years" and 15 "years". This implies that bone age is to some extent a measure of the percentage of a child's growth which has been completed but that all girls do not attain the peak of the adolescent spurt (PHV) when they have completed the same proportion of their total growth, or skeletal maturation.

A similar situation exists in boys. Their skeletal ages are significantly less variable than their chronological ages when they reach 95% of their final stature, but when they reach genital stages 2 or 5, pubic hair stage 3 or the peak of the adolescent growth spurt, the variances of skeletal and chronological age are very similar.

Clearly therefore, a child's skeletal age does not indicate when he or she is likely to reach any stage of sexual development, other than menarche in girls. Skeletal and chronological age, taken together, do provide a basis for predicting approximately when pre-menarcheal girls will experience menarche. The relationship however, is by no means a simple one and we cannot say, for example, that a girl whose skeletal age is two years less than her chronological age will experience menarche two years later than the average, i.e. at 15. This would be possible only if skeletal age were to advance at exactly the average rate from the time of the prediction until the occurrence of menarche and, even then, the variation in skeletal age at menarche, although much less than that at other stages of sexual development, would be sufficient to introduce considerable error.

In practice, a child's skeletal age at any time before her eleventh birthday does not bear a sufficiently close relationship to her age at menarche to be of any value for predictive purposes, although statistically significant correlations have been found from the age of 7 years onwards (Simmons and Greulich, 1943). In girls over the age of 11, prediction is possible but only on the basis of rather complicated statistical procedures which are beyond the scope of this book (Marshall and Limongi, 1976). The practical application of the method is discussed below under the heading "Primary Amenorrhoea".

DISORDERS OF PUBERTY

Delayed Sexual Maturation

If there is no evidence of sexual development by the age of 13·5 yr, in a child of either sex, we must regard the onset of puberty as delayed. The question then arises as to whether this delay is pathological or whether our patient is essentially normal but a late maturer. Delayed puberty is almost invariably associated with short stature and its most common causes are therefore discussed in some detail in Chapter 9. These and other causes are summarized below. It will be clear from this summary that late puberty may be a sign of underlying disease which is potentially far more serious than the absence of sexual development. Careful assessment is therefore essential in all cases.

Slow Tempo of Growth and Maturation. This is usually familial. There are no abnormal findings other than short stature and delayed bone age. The eventual outcome is entirely satisfactory.

Neurological Disorders. The onset of sexual maturation may be delayed by any neurological disorder which impairs the function of the hypothalamo-pituitary axis and hence the production of gonadotrophins. Expert neurological investigation may be necessary to establish the diagnosis in some cases. In others, the diagnosis may be made from the clinical history supported by clinical and biochemical examination. The main demonstrable causes of hypogonadotrophic hypogonadism are:

i) Intracranial space occupying lesions. Craniopharyngiomas or other tumours may prevent secretion of the gonadotrophins by damaging the hypothalamus and/or pituitary.

ii) Inflammation and its sequelae. Encephalitis, meningitis, or granuloma (e.g. sarcoid) may lead to failure of gonadotrophin production. The inflammatory disease itself may have occurred in infancy and may not have been precisely diagnosed even at the time.

iii) Trauma.

iv) Other rare syndromes. Hypogonadism, without obvious cause, may occur either sporadically or in families. It may be associated with anosmia or other congenital abnormalities such as cleft lip and palate or cryptorchidism. In male patients, hypogonadism with cryptorchidism and a small scrotum are features of the Prader–Willi syndrome.

Abnormalities of Pituitary Function. The pituitary may be hypoplastic or aplastic. Also, hypothalamic disorders may result in failure to produce releasing hormones, e.g. luteinizing hormone releasing hormone LHRH or follicle stimulating hormone releasing hormone FSHRH and therefore present clinically as malfunction of the pituitary. There is still controversy as to whether LHRH and FSHRH are separate molecules. In panhypopituitarism, failure to produce growth hormone is accompanied by failure to produce other trophic hormones.

Gonadal Disorders

i) Chromosomal anomalies, e.g. 45XO karyotype - gonadal dysgenesis (Turner's syndrome). Mosaicism in which an X chromosome is absent or defective in one line of cells may also result in defective gonads; 47XYY karyotype, which may be associated with testicular agenesis and 47XXY karyotype – testicular dysgenesis (Klinefelter's syndrome).
ii) Inflammation, e.g. orchitis, as in mumps.
iii) Trauma, bilateral torsion of the ovarian pedicle or the testes may cause atrophy. Rarely, atrophy of the testes may follow bilateral orchidopexy.
iv) Bilateral neoplasms or cysts.

Systemic Illness. Involving the cardiorespiratory, gastrointestinal, urinary or endocrine systems, may inhibit sexual development as well as general somatic growth.

Adverse Environment. Malnutrition, chronic infection and even adverse psychological factors may delay sexual maturation.

Primary Amenorrhoea

Primary amenorrhoea may be associated with normal, absent, or heterosexual development of the secondary sex characteristics.

Absent Sexual Development. The lack of menstruation may be regarded as part of an overall delay of puberty whose causes are discussed above.

Heterosexual Development. Enlargement of the clitoris implies excessive androgen secretion. If the karyotype is normal, the source of the androgens may be a masculinizing tumour of the ovary, an adrenal tumour, or adrenal hyperplasia.

An ovarian tumour will result in high levels of testosterone in the plasma but 17-oxosteroid excretion is likely to be raised only slightly. If the androgen is coming from the adrenal the excretion of 17-oxosteroids is usually significantly raised. For further discussion of this differential diagnosis the reader is referred to standard endocrinology texts or to Dewhurst (1974).

Certain abnormal karyotypes, for example XO/XY mosaicism, may result in heterosexual development and amenorrhoea.

Normal Sexual Development. In these circumstances it may be difficult to decide whether or not the patient should be regarded as suffering from amenorrhoea at all. Age alone is not a criterion, as we have seen earlier. If development of the breasts is proceeding normally, but is incomplete, menarche may yet occur.

Difficulty may arise in the case of the amenarcheal girl with mature or nearly mature breasts. She may also be relatively old (e.g. 17 yr). Is she going to menstruate in due course, or should we regard her as a case of primary amenorrhoea and subject her immediately to all the investigations which this provisional diagnosis implies? If her bone age is already more than 14·5 yr it is unlikely that she will menstruate of her own accord but if her bone age is less than this our problem remains unsolved.

It might be useful to predict the age at which menarche would be most likely to occur in the absence of abnormality, but it would be more useful to estimate the latest age at which a normal child with the same age and bone age as the patient would be likely to experience her first menses. We could then tell our patient (or her parents) that she may remain hopeful of a normal outcome up to that age. However, if she should remain amenarcheal after that time, further action may be necessary. Figure 49 provides the necessary information (Marshall and

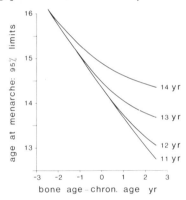

Fig. 49. Age at which menarche will have occurred in 95% of girls who are premenarcheal at given values of (Bone Age — Chronological Age). Separate lines apply to girls of different chronological ages as indicated. Reproduced from Marshall and Limongi (1976) with permission.

Limongi 1976). To use it, we subtract the patient's bone age from her chronological age and take a perpendicular from this value on the x-axis to the line marked with the chronological age nearest to that of the patient. The "95% limit" of her age at menarche may then be read on the y-axis. This limit is the age at which menarche will have occurred in 95% of girls who have the patient's bone age at her present chronological age. Thus, if the patient reaches this limit without experiencing menarche, there is only a 5% chance that her develop-ment is normal.

uterus is functioning normally but

the genital tract is imperforate at some point. If the hymen is imperforate, with accumulated blood above it, this may be clearly seen on inspection of the vulva. At other times the blockage may be less obvious. This is a matter for a gynaecologist.

Absence of the uterus may be associated with absence of the vagina in otherwise normal females but also occurs in androgen insensitivity (testicular feminization). Patients with testicular feminization have a male (46 XY) karyotype. At adolescence the breasts and bodily configuration develop in the normal female pattern but sexual hair is usually scanty or absent. The testes may be intra-abdominal, in the inguinal canal, or in the labia. The plasma values of testosterone are usually within the normal male range. Sometimes, patients are unusually tall by female standards although their stature seldom exceeds the normal male range.

Isosexual Precocious Puberty

Puberty may be considered precocious if the secondary sex characters begin to develop before the 8th birthday in girls and slightly later e.g. 8·5 to 9 yr in boys.

True Sexual Precocity. In this condition, sexual development is entirely normal apart from the fact that it occurs at an unusually early age. In about 85% of girls and 65% of boys the cause is unknown (idiopathic precocious puberty), although in very early cases a recognizable organic cause is found more frequently. The commonest cause is an abnormality of the central nervous system. This may be congenital but may also be the result of infection (encephalitis or meningitis), trauma or neoplasm.

Precocious puberty may occur in polyostotic fibrous dysplasia, which is otherwise characterized by bone lesions and cafe au lait spots. It sometimes occurs in hyperthyroidism and in hypothyroidism.

Pseudoprecocious Puberty. This is precocious sexual development occurring independently of the normal regulating mechanisms. The cause may be a tumour e.g. chorionepithelioma, or an extragonadal teratoma secreting a substance with gonadotrophic properties. Some tumours of the ovary or testis may secrete sex hormones without gonadotrophic stimulation.

Ingestion of oestrogen (e.g. mother's contraceptive pills) may cause isosexual precocious puberty in girls.

In boys, excessive androgen secretion by the adrenal may cause isosexual precocity associated with infantile testes, as in congenital adrenal hyperplasia. A virilizing adenoma or carcinoma of the adrenal will have the same effect. Adrenal tumours rarely cause isosexual precocity in girls.

Incomplete Isosexual Precocity. This term refers to either precocious development of the breasts (premature thelarche) or to premature growth of the pubic or axillary hair (premature pubarche), in the absence of the other. Premature thelarche may be due to hypersensitivity of the breast to normal amounts of circulating oestrogen but this is by no means certain. The cause of premature pubarche is not yet fully understood.

Heterosexual Precocious Puberty

This results from exposure to excessive amounts of the gonadal hormones appropriate to the opposite sex. The cause in girls may be an arrhenoblastoma of the ovary; congential adrenal hyperplasia; an adrenal tumour; a teratoma or administration of androgen. In boys, the condition may result from a feminizing tumour of the adrenal, a teratoma, or ingestion of oestrogens. Adolescent gynaecomastia occurs frequently in patients with Klinefelter's syndrome (XXY karyotype).

5

Maturity and its Measurement

INTRODUCTION

We have seen in the preceding chapters that all normal children follow very similar patterns of physical development. The post-natal growth pattern is remarkably constant, for example in stature, which has a high initial velocity but constant deceleration until the adolescent spurt begins. The cartilagenous parts of the skeleton become calcified and the developing calcium deposits undergo changes in shape which are common to all normal subjects and which can be studied radiologically. Finally, all normal children experience at some time the complex of physiological and anatomical changes which we call puberty. However, children vary greatly in the rate at which they pass through these changes and in the age at which they are completed. Therefore, children of the same chronological age vary in their progress towards adulthood and have different quanta of growth and development to complete before we would describe them as "grown-ups". In other words, they differ in their physical maturity.

For example, a perfectly healthy 13-year-old girl might not have experienced any of the changes of puberty. X-rays of her skeleton might show that the centres of ossification were not yet as fully calcified as they are in most other girls of that age. She would probably be small by comparison with her peers because she had not yet experienced the

86

adolescent growth spurt. In contrast, one of her friends, also aged 13, might have completed her sexual development, begun to menstruate and almost reached her final stature.

Differences of maturity are usually most obvious between the ages of 10 and 13 when early maturers are undergoing all the changes of puberty and are strikingly different in size and general appearance from the late maturers in whom these changes have not begun. However, comparable differences in maturity exist throughout childhood. Two 6-year-olds may have the same stature but one of them may be destined to experience an early puberty and stop growing early. The other may reach puberty later, continue to grow for longer, and be taller as an adult.

DEFINING MATURITY

The first difficulty we meet in attempting to measure a child's maturity is the lack of any satisfactory or generally accepted unit of measurement. We cannot use units of length, such as centimetres, or units of time, such as years, because the process of maturation is not completed in everyone by the attainment of the same amount of linear growth or by the passage of any fixed amount of time.

In order to be valid, a measure of maturity must be based on a maturational process whose end point is known in advance. This implies that it has the same final value or state in every person. To be clinically useful it must also pass through essentially the same sequence of clearly recognizable stages in each individual. Ideally, we would require something like a hundred stages, with the attainment of each one representing an equal step towards the final mature state. We would then be able to say, for example, this child reached stage 56, therefore he is 56% mature. Unfortunately, no such ideal scale of maturation is available.

There are, however, individual processes, for example, growth in stature, which do reach a recognizable end point. Thus, if we had a chart showing repeated measurements of a single individual's stature from early childhood until he had grown up, we could tell at what age ⋯ when he had attained, ⋯ of view,

aware of this because, at that stage, adult stature was going to be.

Thus, although stature may be used retrospectively to study the maturation of individuals after they have become adults, it is of no value at all in assessing maturity during childhood. A 7-year-old who has the same stature as the average child of 6 is sometimes said to have a "height age" of 6, but this does not necessarily mean that his maturity is that of an average 6-year-old. It means only that his stature is at the 50th centile for 6-year-olds and this is just another way of saying that his stature is at the 10th centile for a 7-year-old, i.e. that he is rather small for his age. His "height age" does not tell us whether he is short because he is a late maturer who will eventually reach an adult stature higher than the 10th centile, or whether he is destined to finish up at, or below, this centile. For the same reasons weight and "weight age" are not valid measures of maturity.

Unfortunately all the criteria used for measuring maturity have disadvantages. Nevertheless some are more satisfactory than others. Skeletal, sexual and dental development have been studied most fully.

SKELETAL DEVELOPMENT

The development of the skeleton provides one of the most useful indices of maturity, and the one most closely related to growth in stature. As the cartilage of the growing skeleton is gradually converted to bone, the calcified tissue in each centre of ossification undergoes changes of shape and size which can be observed radiographically. The sequence of changes exhibited by each centre is remarkably constant and varies only in minor details from one child to another. When all the centres are fully calcified, the skeleton is mature. Thus, skeletal maturation fulfils the essential criteria for an adequate scale of maturity, i.e. it reaches a common end point in all adults whose growth is completed and passes through a number of recognizable changes which are common to all children.

TECHNIQUES OF ASCERTAINING SKELETAL MATURITY

Most authors have, in principle, divided the process of calcification in each ossification centre into a series of stages and then combined the stages reached by each bone in some way, to give a measure of a child's skeletal maturity. However, as some of the stages are difficult to recognize, a certain amount of observer error is inevitable.

Some authors have tried to minimize this error by using as stages only the beginning or completion of ossification in skeletal centres, or the fusion and lack of fusion of epiphyses. However, any method which uses only the appearance of centres and the fusion of epiphyses is inefficient because it neglects a great deal of information which might be obtained by studying the intermediate stages in the development of each bone. Also, in order to obtain a reasonably accurate assessment of skeletal age in this way, it is necessary to study a large number of centres throughout the body and hence extensive radiography is required. If intermediate stages are also used it is necessary only to X-ray a small area, such as the hand and wrist, which contain a variety of bones, each providing a sequence of changes appropriate to our purpose. The radius, ulna, and carpal bones, together with the metacarpals and phalanges of the first, third and fifth digits total 20 bones suitable for study. Each of these bones has its own sequence of changes, so that progress can be seen in at least one of them at almost every stage of development.

The knee and the hip have also been studied from this point of view, but it is impossible to shield the ovaries adequately from radiation while X-raying the hip and this region is therefore unsuitable for routine work in girls. For practical purposes, the hand and wrist is the most suitable region and is nowadays almost the only one used in the clinical assessment of skeletal development.

Greulich and Pyle Technique

The best-known technique is that based on the "atlas" method of Greulich and Pyle (1959). This "atlas" consists of a series of radiographs which are thought to be typical of children at some 30 different points along the maturity scale. The illustrations were selected by examining serial radiographs of healthy children from prosperous homes in Cleveland, Ohio. The films from each age group were arranged in order so that one bone increased progressively in maturity. The central film, i.e. the one showing the median maturity for that bone, was ——————— ——— of the given bone in the age group. ——— An

logical ——

The method of using the atlas is to ——— well as possible, with one of the illustrations in the book. The skeletal attributed to the illustration which most closely resembles the patient's radiograph is the skeletal age of the patient. The matching process is necessarily subjective and this is one weakness of the technique.

Another problem is that the patient's radiograph frequently does not exactly match any of the standards. Some bones may be more advanced, and others less so, than those illustrated in the most appropriate standard. The atlas does suggest a method for assigning bone ages to individual bones so that, by some kind of averaging procedure, it is possible to establish a bone age for the child. This method is seldom used however and presents theoretical difficulties.

A more fundamental objection to the atlas method is that each standard radiograph is said to represent a "bone age" equal to the chronological age of the child on whom it was based. The system therefore measures maturity in units of age. This is unsatisfactory because any scale of maturity based on age has two fundamental weaknesses. Firstly, it is impossible to assign an age to an individual whose bones are fully mature and, secondly, the average chronological age at which children reach a given stage of maturation may vary between one population and another. For example, we might use a method similar to that by which the Greulich and Pyle Atlas was compiled to determine the appearance of the hand and wrist radiograph in a typical 12-year-old. This would represent a bone age of 12 "years" and it would be correct to say that the average bone age of 12-year-old children was 12 "years". What then would happen if we used our new standard to study a population who were about a year advanced in their rate of maturation? We should discover that our so-called "12 year" standard was representative of the average 11-year-old in the second population. This leads to an ambiguous deduction such as "the average bone age of 11-year-old children in the population is 12 years".

It would therefore be more satisfactory if a maturity scale were defined without reference to age. Each individual would be given a number of "points" which would describe his maturity status in much the same way as we might describe his height in centimetres but with the important difference that the final score achieved at maturity would be the same in everybody. Children who had not yet reached maturity would exhibit a wide range of scores and it would be possible to create standards giving the mean and centiles of maturity scores at each age. These would be similar in principle to the centile standards for height and weight although, as we shall see below, the curves would be quite different in shape.

The TW2 Method

One way of constructing a suitable maturity scale would be to allot a numerical score to each stage of the development of each bone in, for example, the hand and wrist. An overall score would then be obtained by some kind of averaging process. This approach is adopted in the "TW2" technique (Tanner *et al.*, 1975a). In developing this technique, Tanner *et al.* examined a number of longitudinal series of radiographs, taken every six months over several years, of the hands and wrists of normal British children. They studied successive changes in the shape and density of the margins of each centre of ossification from the time at which it first became visible, as a speck of calcium, until it developed its adult appearance. They divided the continuous development of each bone into a number of discrete stages which could be described without ambiguity by verbal criteria and illustrated by drawings. Figure 50 illustrates the stages for the first metacarpal. A corresponding sequence of stages occurred in any given bone in the serial radiographs of all the children in the study.

The radius, metacarpals, phalanges, hamate and trapezium each have nine stages and the ulna and the remaining carpal bones each have eight. The stages are defined by letters A B C D etc. and stage A means that the bone is not yet visible. The same stages are used for boys and girls and for all ethnic groups so far examined.

Each stage of each bone was given a numerical score, which was determined after making due allowance for the difference in the contribution to overall maturity made by the various bones i.e. a bone which reached its mature state earlier than most would make a small contribution to overall maturity and its scores would be correspondingly low.

In fact, three separate scoring systems were derived. One involved the carpals only; another included the radius, ulna and finger bones (henceforth called "RUS", meaning radius, ulna and short bones) while the third (20 bone score) combined these groups. In all cases the final, or adult, score is 1,000 points. The theoretical basis of the scoring

scores were calculated, it was found that the two sexes differed systematically. This was particularly so in the group of bones including the radius, ulna, metacarpals and phalanges. This situation arises because, although all the bones mature earlier in girls than in boys, some are very early and others are less so.

Since girls and boys have different scores for the same stages, two radiographs identical in appearance but taken from a boy and a girl,

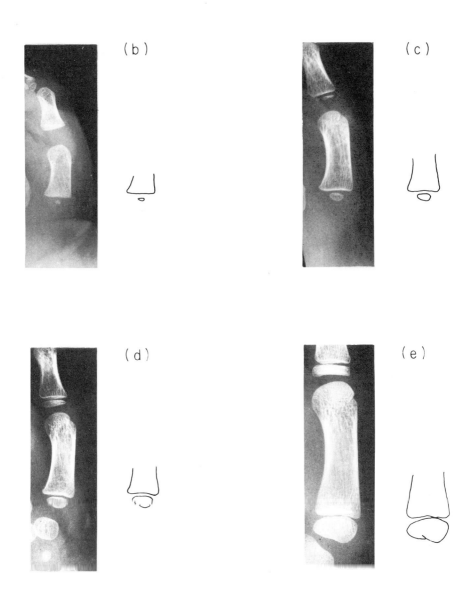

(a)

Fig. 50 (a and b). Stages of ossification of the epiphysis of the first metacarpal (TW2 method). Based on Tanner *et al.* (1975).

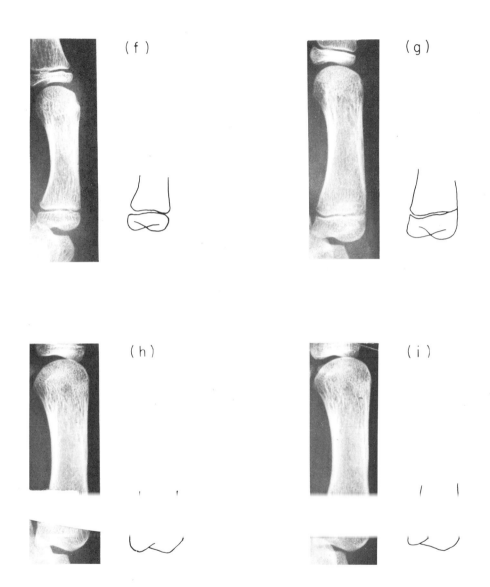

(f)

(g)

(h)

(i)

(b)

Fig. 50

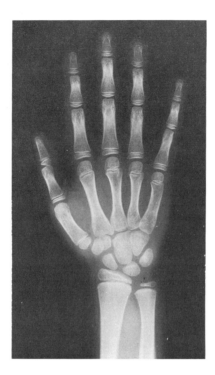

Fig. 51. Radiograph of hand and wrist positioned for assessment of skeletal maturity by the TW2 method.

would be given different overall scores and would not represent the same maturity. Theoretically, however, radiographs of a boy and a girl which merited the same scores, although they would not look the same, would represent comparable degrees of maturation.

Standards for TW2 Maturity Scores. Knowledge of a child's maturity score is useless unless there are some standards of normality with which we can compare it. The most appropriate standards give the mean and centiles of the maturity scores attained by radiographs of children at given ages in just the same way as we might use the mean and centiles of their statures. These standards, of course, just like height standards, are strictly valid only for the population on which they are based although, as far as we know, the basic rating and scoring system is of universal validity.

An example of these standards is shown in Fig. 52. On this chart, the scores on the vertical scale are divided by ten, so that the maximum is 100 and not 1,000 points. The scale is non-linear, because it has been modified mathematically to keep the centiles apart at the two ends,

TABLE VI

Calculation of bone ages based on X-ray shown in Fig. 51
of girl aged 8·031

Bone		Stage	INDIVIDUAL BONE SCORES		
			20-Bone	RUS	Carpal
Radius		G	85	114	
Ulna		E	39	45	
	1	E	18	24	
Metacarpal	3	F	17	23	
	5	E	12	17	
	1	E	14	20	
Proximal	3	E	13	19	
Phalanx	5	E	13	18	
Middle	3	E	13	18	
Phalanx	5	E	14	18	
	1	E	15	22	
Distal	3	E	10	15	
Phalanx	5	E	11	15	
Capitate		H	113		203
Hamate		G	85		161
Triquetral		F	36		80
Lunate		F	35		84
Scaphoid		E	29		71
Trapezium		F	32		80
Trapezoid		G	40		97
	SCORE		644	388	776
	BONE AGE		8·91	8·84	9·13

Fig. 52. Centiles of TW2 (RUS) bone scores in British boys. For explanation of interrupted lines and relationship of bone score to bone age, see text. Reproduced from Marshall (1975) with permission.

there they would otherwise be crowded. The standard centile curves can be used in the same way as stature centiles, so that we can say, for example, that a boy, aged 10 with a maturity score of 30 is at the 50th centile for RUS skeletal maturity. This would mean that 50% of boys of his age were less mature than he while 50% were more mature. If his bone score were far below the 10th centile this would indicate a delay which was sufficiently unusual to merit investigation lest there be a pathological cause. A score above the 50th centile implies advanced maturity and one above the 90th centile is sufficiently advanced to arouse suspicion.

The curves may also be used to convert the score into a "bone age". This is the age at which the 50th centile score equals the child's actual score. For example, a boy with an RUS score of 300 (see Fig. 52 where this score is represented as 30), has a skeletal age of 10 yr, whatever his chronological age may be. In practice, this conversion is made by means of tables which are given with the standards. Charts and tables are also available for calculating skeletal ages on the basis of carpal or total (20 bone) scores. However, for most practical purposes, including the prediction of adult height, the carpal bones do not contribute useful information. Therefore, only the RUS score and bone age need be calculated in most clinical work.

Some paediatricians consider the TW2 method of Tanner *et al.* (1975a) to be too laborious for clinical use because it is necessary to examine each bone in turn with some care. However, the same care is required if the bone age is to be estimated accurately using the atlas of Greulich and Pyle. The apparent simplicity of the latter method makes it easy to use without due care and this may lead to very inaccurate results. The necessity to give a score to each bone, as in the TW2 method, precludes a slovenly approach.

PREDICTION OF ADULT HEIGHT

Relationship of Child's Final Height to Parents' Height

When a child grows up under favourable conditions, the final stature he attains is largely dependent on heredity and may therefore be predicted approximately from the heights of his parents. In other words the child of a tall parent is likely to be a tall child and the child of short parents is likely to be short. However, the relationship between this "mid-parent height" and the child's ultimate stature is not close enough for a prediction based solely upon it to be of much value for practical purposes.

Relationship of Child's Height to his own Adult Height

As an alternative to using the parents' heights we might try to predict
the child's adult stature from his own stature at any given age. This
approach is not at all satisfactory for children less than three years old.
The length of the newborn baby reflects chiefly the conditions he
experienced *in utero* and the true relationship of the child's height to
his own eventual adult stature is not established until about age 3.
After this age it is possible to predict the child's adult height from his
current stature although the prediction is not sufficiently accurate to be
of much value for practical purposes. The accuracy can be increased in
girls over the age of 6, and in boys more than 8 if some allowance is
made for the variation of maturity in children belonging to each age
group.

A child's height at any given age depends not only on the final stature
to which his growth is directed but also on the proportion of his growth
which has been completed. If we could measure this proportion accurately we would be able to make a correspondingly accurate prediction of adult height. We cannot measure this directly in a child who is
still growing and we must make use of his maturity in some other aspect
of development, which we can measure, and which bears a meaningful
relationship to his stature. "Bone age" is the most useful criterion
available to us at the present time.

Role of "Bone Age" in Height Prediction

The tables of Bayley and Pinneau (1952), for use with the Gruelich and
Pyle skeletal maturity standards, are the most widely used basis for predicting adult height at the time of writing. There are three separate
tables: one to be used when bone age is retarded for more than a year,
the second if bone age is within one year of the chronological age and the
third when bone age is advanced by more than a year. Each table gives
the percentage of mature height attained at each age by children in
whom the relationship of bone age to chronological age is appropriate
to that table. The prediction is made from this percentage and the
child's known stature at the time. However, the exact bone age cannot
be taken into account and therefore, even if there were a precise
relationship between bone age and the amount of growth completed,
the tables could not be very accurate. The tables cover only the age
range from 8 years upwards.

The development of the TW2 method of estimating bone age has
provided a new basis for predicting adult height which permits a

quantitative allowance for any degree of skeletal maturity in children over 4 years of age. The prediction is made by working out an equation of the form

$$\text{"predicted adult height"} = \frac{A \times \text{present height (cm)} + B \times \text{chronological age (yr)} + C \times \text{bone age (yr)} + D.}$$

The tables of Tanner et al. (1975b) give the values of the coefficients A, B, C and D for children of different ages. There is a separate equation for each half year of chronological age and for pre- and post-menarcheal girls aged from 11 to 14. In order to use these tables the bone age must be calculated by the TW2 method, using the standards described earlier in this chapter and omitting the carpal bones, i.e. using the RUS bone age. The only other information we require is the child's stature, which must be accurately measured and preferably within two weeks of the day on which the hand was X-rayed. The girl whose radiograph is shown in Fig. 51 was 8 years old with a stature of 125·7 cm. Her RUS bone age as 8·84 yr. The tables give the following values for the coefficients in the prediction equation

$$A = 0 \cdot 92 \quad B = -4 \cdot 4 \quad C = -1 \cdot 5 \quad D = 95.$$

Therefore her predicted adult height is

$$0 \cdot 92 \times 125 \cdot 7 - 4 \cdot 4 \times 8 \cdot 031 - 1 \cdot 5 \times 8 \cdot 84 + 95 = 162 \cdot 04 \text{ cm.}$$

Predictions made by this method are not always as accurate as one might like but they are the best available and the technique has the great advantage that its range of possible error is known. Boys aged between 4 and 13 are predicted to within ± 7 cm of their true adult height in 95% of cases and this range falls to ± 6 cm at 14 and then progressively to $\pm 1 \cdot 6$ cm at age 17·5. Girls aged between 4 and 11 are subject to the same errors as boys. The 95% confidence limits in pre-menarcheal girls aged between 12 and 13 are ± 5 and ± 4 cm respectively while in post-menarcheal girls of the same ages the limits are ± 4 and ± 3 cm respectively. The smallest range of error ($\pm 1 \cdot 5$ cm) is reached at age 15. The prediction may be improved slightly by applying a "parental correction". Tanner et al. (1975b) suggest taking the average of the two parents' statures and subtracting 167 cm from it, one-third of the answer is then added to the predicted stature. This correction may not be valid in all cases and further work may show that the allowance for parental height should change in relation to the child's maturity.

Strictly speaking, the height prediction equations are valid only for children who are within the same normal limits for height and bone age as the children whose measurements and radiographs were used to calculate them. This limitation also applies to the Bayley/Pinneau method. Caution is therefore necessary in applying either method to children who are unusually tall or short and to those who are greatly advanced or retarded in bone age. The validity of the method as applied to children of races other than Caucasian has not been tested.

There are two clinical situations in which an accurate prediction of adult height would be particularly valuable. Firstly, there is the problem of very tall boys and girls. Here prediction would help us to decide whether or not hormone treatment should be given and in assessing its effectiveness (see Chapter 10). Roche and Wettenhall (1969) used the Bayley/Pinneau tables to predict the adult height of 29 untreated tall girls. In fact only seven of these were above the 97th centile and they were, on average, over-predicted by only 0·7 cm. Zachmann *et al.* (1975) found that the mean final stature of nine tall girls was 0·37 cm less than the mean predicted value (TW2 method). It is therefore probable, although it has not yet been established, that the final statures of most tall girls would be predicted by the Tanner/Whitehouse (TW2) method with an accuracy similar to that obtained with subjects whose statures are within the normal range.

Secondly, there are the small, but essentially normal children whose shortness is due to delayed maturation. The available evidence indicates that the predictions based on the TW2 method are sufficiently accurate, when applied to late maturing, but otherwise normal children, to provide valid grounds for reassuring them as to their future growth prospects. Neither the Bayley/Pinneau nor the TW2 method of height prediction is valid when applied to children whose smallness has a clear pathological origin as in chondrodystrophies, endocrine disorder, renal disease etc.

PUBERTY AS A MATURITY INDICATOR

The events of puberty are discussed in detail in Chapter 4. Here we shall summarize briefly their relationship to other aspects of the child's development.

The development of the secondary sex characteristics is associated with the adolescent growth spurt. Therefore a child of any age, who has no endocrine abnormality but is without sexual development, has yet to experience the spurt. A boy in early puberty also has the spurt before him but this is not necessarily true of girls, some of whom reach peak height velocity while they are still in breast stage 2.

Menarche nearly always occurs shortly after peak height velocity, therefore it is a reasonable working assumption that the growth of any post-menarcheal girl has begun to slow down towards its final halt. Most girls experience menarche when their bone ages are between 12·5 and 14·5 yr. The bone age of a pre-menarcheal girl may be used to predict approximately when her menarche will occur. This prediction however is dependent upon complex statistical arguments which are beyond the scope of this book (see Marshall and Limongi, 1976). A simple prediction based on the argument "this girl's bone age is delayed by e.g. one year, therefore she will experience menarche a year later than average", would not be valid.

There is little relationship between the maturation of the skeleton and the beginning of puberty in either sex. The bone age at which the breasts develop in girls or the genitalia begin to develop in boys varies just as much as their chronological ages (Marshall, 1974a). A pre-pubertal child whose bone age is advanced, but within the normal range of variation, will not necessarily experience an early puberty. Similarly, a delayed bone age does not necessarily imply late puberty. Very early (precocious) puberty is associated with an advanced bone age and the bone age of a child who will experience puberty extremely late is usually delayed. When skeletal maturation is very retarded as in growth hormone deficiency, puberty does not usually occur until the bone age is within the range at which puberty begins in normal children. The actual chronological ages of the growth hormone deficient children are, of course, much greater than their bone ages.

DENTAL MATURITY

The dentition may be called "mature" when all the secondary teeth (with the possible exception of the third molar) are fully erupted. This state is reached with the same number of mature teeth in nearly all normal individuals. Dental development therefore fulfils the basic criterion of a maturity indicator i.e. it has the same end-point in all normal subjects. Also, during its development, each tooth passes through a series of stages which are the same in all children and can be studied radiographically.

There are many techniques for assessing dental maturity or "dental age". They vary in complexity from simply counting the number of erupted teeth to radiographic methods which give "scores" to stages of development for different teeth. The most advanced of these methods is similar in principle to the Tanner/Whitehouse method of estimating bone age (Demirjian et al., 1973). However, a child's dental maturity does not apparently bear a constant relationship to other aspects of development, such as bone age or stature, although Filipsson and Hall (1975) have recently shown that it is possible to predict a child's adult stature from her age and stature at the time when certain teeth erupt.

RELATIONSHIP BETWEEN DIFFERENT MEASURES OF MATURATION

It is clear from the above discussions that all aspects of the child's maturation do not necessarily proceed at the same rate. There is therefore no satisfactory measurement of the child's overall maturity. We must consider the maturation of different systems entirely separately and direct our attention to the system which is most relevant in a given context, e.g. to the maturation of the skeleton when we wish to predict adult height.

Sexual maturation is an important index of endocrine function in older children and has some relationship to overall growth.

The relationship between dental development and other measures of maturity can be of interest in some clinical situations. In hypothyroidism, the development of both the skeleton and the teeth is retarded. However, in precocious puberty, the accelerated skeletal and sexual maturation which occurs is not usually accompanied by a corresponding advancement in the dentition. In progeria, the bone age may be normal but the dental development retarded.

6

Body Composition and Growth of Individual Tissues

INTRODUCTION

From the time of conception onwards, the growing organism is constantly changing, not only in size and shape, but in the relative amounts of the different types of cells and tissues which make up its total structure. The quantitative relationships between the different components of the total body mass are the subject of studies in body composition.

EMBRYO AND FOETUS

The fertilized ovum does not increase in size whilst the earliest cell divisions are taking place and the cells therefore become progressively smaller with each division. By about the ninth day, when the blastocyst has implanted in the uterine wall, the cells have begun to enlarge before they divide and the divisions have become staggered so that only a few cells divide at any one time.

Extracellular fluid probably appears at about the time of implantation. Fluid passes from the uterine cavity through the outer cells of the embryo, which act as a dialysing membrane, into the intercellular spaces between the inner cell mass and the outer cells. Nutrients can only reach the inner cells through the extracellular fluid which is therefore essential for further growth.

Towards the end of the first month, the primitive connective tissue cells, in the regions which will eventually form the skeleton, become more closely packed and lay down a matrix between themselves. This is the primitive cartilage which begins to ossify during the second month of foetal life. Before ossification begins, there is very little calcium in the foetus but the amount increases rapidly from the eighth week onwards as the bones grow and become more fully calcified.

In early gestation the organism contains no fat other than the essential lipids in the central nervous system and phospholipids in the cell walls. During the first half of gestation the foetus contains less than $0\cdot5\%$ fat. After this, white fat begins to appear in the connective tissue cells under the skin and in the omenta while brown adipose tissue occurs around the neck and between the scapulae. By 28 weeks the foetus is about $3\cdot5\%$ fat; at 34 weeks $7\cdot5\%$ and a full term baby of $3\cdot5$ kg is about 16% fat.

Very young foetuses, weighing about 1 g contain about 95% water, (i.e. a higher percentage than is found in adult human plasma) but the amount of water in the fat free tissue falls throughout gestation and, at term, water accounts for only 82% of the fat free weight, and about 69% of total weight. However, the newborn still has a much higher water content than the adult in whom water is only 72% of the fat free weight.

Information about the body composition of the foetus has been obtained by chemical analysis but there is practically no direct analytical evidence about the changes in body composition after birth. Indirect methods have been applied to living children at different ages.

CHILDHOOD AND ADOLESCENCE

Body Fat

Total amount. Several techniques exist by which we can establish the amount of fat in the body after birth.

The density of the body decreases as its fat content rises because fat is less dense than the other components of the tissues. It is therefore possible to calculate the percentage of fat in a living subject if his body density is known. This can be measured by weighing him first in air and then in water.

Density = weight ÷ volume.

Volume in litres = (weight in air — weight when completely sub-
merged in water) in kg.

When the subject is being weighed under water he sits or lies on a
frame of known density which is suspended from a spring balance. The
weight recorded must be corrected for residual air in the lungs, therefore the subject breathes out as much as possible before immersion and
as soon as he surfaces he breathes from a bag containing oxygen. The
dilution of this oxygen with nitrogen and carbon dioxide provides a
measure of the residual air. The formula generally used for calculating
fat from body density is

$$\text{percent fat} = \left(\frac{4 \cdot 95}{\text{density}} - 4 \cdot 5 \right) \times 100 \ (\text{Siri, 1956}).$$

Useful measurements are only possible if the subject is not frightened
by the immersion process. The technique is therefore unsuitable for use
with small children but can be applied successfully to older children and
adults. Durnin and Rohaman (1967) studied 48 adolescent boys and 38
girls. They found a mean density of 1·065, corresponding to 15·9%
body fat for the boys and of 1·045, i.e. 24% body fat for the girls.

Another measure of body fat is the difference between the lean body
mass, (i.e. the estimated mass of the body deprived of all fat) and total
body weight. This method is easier to apply to children, but as we shall
see below, the estimation of lean body mass is itself subject to error. The
values for percentages of body fat shown in Fig. 53 were obtained in
this way. They show a startling difference between the two sexes. In
boys, the percentage of fat reaches a maximum about the age of 10, i.e.
before puberty, and then falls. In girls the percentage is at its lowest
at about age 7 and then rises at a steady rate until 14. This means that
50th centile girls aged 13 have nearly twice as much fat as 50th centile
boys of the same age. A thin (10th centile) 16-year-old girl has about the
same percentage of fat in her body as an obese (90th centile) 16-year-
old boy.

Measurements of skinfold thickness (Tanner and Whitehouse, 1975)
and radiographic measurements of the thickness of the subcutaneous
fat reflect changes in total body fat and allow the relative fatness of
different individuals to be compared with an accuracy sufficient for
many purposes. Both these techniques have the advantage that they
are suitable for clinical use and they can be used to estimate the amount
of fat at specified sites. The triceps and subscapular skinfold thicknesses
in both sexes increase up to the age of about nine months, after which
they decrease gradually for about the next seven years. In boys, there is

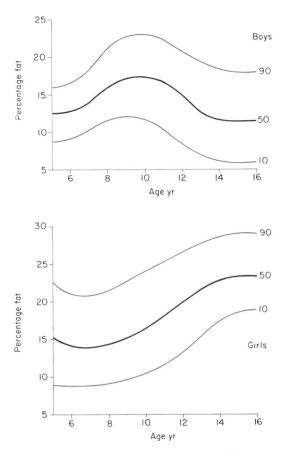

Fig. 53. Centiles of percentage of body fat in boys and girls at different ages. Based on data from Rauh and Schumsky (1968).

a brief increase in the fat of the limbs before the adolescent growth spurt and then a fall as indicated by the triceps skinfold, although the subscapular skinfold continues to increase (Fig. 54). Adolescent girls gain fat at both sites and continue to do so until adulthood. This description is, of course, a generalized one and individuals vary greatly in the pattern of change in their skinfold thickness.

The changes in thickness of subcutaneous fat during childhood are shown more precisely by radiographic data (Tanner, 1965). Figure 55 shows the rate of increase in subcutaneous fat measured on radiographs of three sites on the calf, arm and thigh. Data from the three sites are combined and the time scale is given in years before and after peak height velocity instead of chronological age, so that we can see the

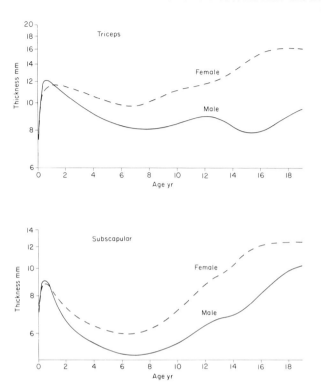

Fig. 54. 50th centiles of triceps and subscapular skinfold thickness in boys and girls at different ages. Based on data from Tanner and Whitehouse (1975).

relationship of the fat changes to puberty, regardless of the age at which this occurs in different subjects. The rate of fat gain drops during the adolescent growth spurt in both sexes but, in girls, the value remains positive, i.e. they continue to gain fat although they do so more slowly. In boys, on the other hand, the rate of gain becomes negative, i.e. they actually lose fat from the sites examined. After PHV, as growth in stature slows down, the rate of gain in fat increases again in both sexes.

Obesity and the Structure of Adipose Tissue. At birth, only 45% of the weight of adipose tissue is due to fat. Water accounts for 46% and protein for most of the remainder. By the age of six months the proportion of water has fallen to 27% and fat has risen to 60% (Baker, G. T., 1969).

An increase of fat in the body may be due to either an increase in the number of fat-containing cells, or the enlargement of existing cells. In order to decide which of these processes is more important we must be able to estimate the number of cells present. Two methods are used

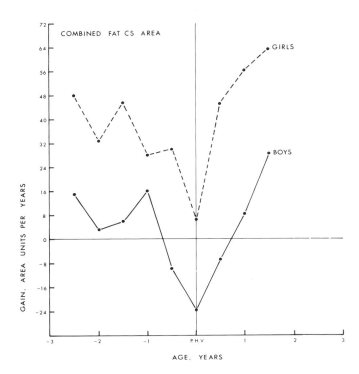

Fig. 55. Rate of increase in thickness of subcutaneous fat. Data combined from radiographs at three sites, on the calf, thigh and arm. Reproduced from Tanner (1965) with permission.

for counting cells in adipose tissue. The first is to remove the collagen with the help of an enzyme (collagenase), fix the fat in the cells with osmium tetroxide and then suspend them in glycerol. They can then be counted electronically. The second is to cut frozen sections from the tissue and count the cells under the microscope.

A cell will only be counted by either method if it contains some fat. Cells which are capable of holding fat but are empty will not be counted. The amount of fat in a given volume of tissue is determined chemically on a separate sample and this value is divided by the number of cells in the same volume giving an estimate of the average amount of lipid per cell. This is taken as a measure of mean cell size.

Brook, *et al.* (1972) estimated the number of cells with fat in the bodies of 64 children who were not obese and 52 who were obese. The number of fat-containing cells apparently increased five times between the ages of one and 13 years. Although girls are fatter than boys they do not appear to have a greater number of cells and must therefore have more fat in each cell. Children who had become obese during their first year of life had more cells with fat in them than children of average weight. This was not true, however, of those who become fat later in childhood although the total amount of fat in the body was similar in the two obese groups. Thus, obesity can be achieved without an unusually high number of fat cells by increasing the fat content of each cell and the number of fat cells may be of no great importance in the aetiology of obesity.

Brown and White Adipose Tissue. The specialized form of adipose tissue known as "brown adipose tissue" is capable of producing heat in response to cold exposure. It is not involved in the formation, storage and supply of fatty acids, which are the main functions of white adipose tissue. The production of heat by white adipose tissue is only a by-product of its metabolic activity and no additional release of heat as a specific response has been demonstrated. In the new-born child, thermogenesis in brown adipose tissue plays an important part in regulating the body temperature. The main deposits of brown adipose tissue are in the region of the arteries in the neck, extending into the mediastinum and below the clavicle to the axilla. It may also be found in the posterior peritoneum and round the kidneys. Although brown adipose tissue persists into adult life, its thermogenic function declines with age and its role in the adult is not yet clear.

Lean Body Mass and its Components

Estimation from Total Body Water. If it is assumed that fat does not contain any water, and that the percentage of water in the remainder of the body is constant from one individual to another then we can estimate the weight of the fat free body (lean body mass) by measuring how much water it contains. It is usually assumed for this purpose that the fat free body of the adult contains 73·2% water. However, there is good evidence that the amount of water in the lean body mass does, in fact, vary between individuals and therefore the body water does not accurately reflect the lean body mass. It does, however, provide a basis for comparing groups of subjects in whom it can be assumed that the mean content of water in the lean body mass is approximately constant. Total body water may be measured by dilution techniques using antipyrene, urea, alcohol, tritium and deuterium oxide.

The percentage of water in the body falls during gestation and for the first month or so of post-natal life. However, by the time body weight reaches 7 or 8 kg the percentage of water is usually within the adult range. The water content of adults varies between about 55 to 70% of the total body weight, as distinct from the lean body mass. After the age of about 4, boys have a higher body water content in relation to body weight than girls because the boys are less fat and their lean body mass is a greater proportion of their body weight.

The total body water is made up of extracellular and intracellular portions, often referred to as "compartments", the proportions of which change considerably in early life. The extracellular water can be estimated by measuring the dilution of thiosulphate which diffuses throughout this compartment but not into the cells. According to Friis-Hansen (1957) approximately 45% of the total body weight of a full term baby is due to extracellular water which accounts for about 65% of the total body water. The proportion of extracellular water decreases after birth and is only about 30% of the body weight when the body reaches 5 kg. The intracellular water increases during childhood from about 35% of the body weight at birth to about 47% between the ages of 7 and 16 years.

Estimation from Potassium ^{40}K. Another indirect measure of lean body mass can be made by detecting and counting gamma rays emitted by potassium ^{40}K which is always present in the body. The technique requires a whole body counter, which is a chamber shielded against background radiation and fitted with scintillators to detect gamma rays. The method is harmless and can be applied to small children.

The percentage of potassium, in relation to body weight, falls during the first six months of life as the percentage of fat in the body rises and the lean body mass becomes a smaller fraction of the whole but, after this, the potassium increases (Maresh and Groome, 1966). From five years onwards, boys have more potassium than girls of the same weight which is in keeping with the greater percentage of fat in girls.

The use of body potassium to calculate lean body mass depends upon the assumption that the concentration of potassium in the lean body mass, and the proportion of this which is radioactive, remain constant. It is, however, very doubtful whether this condition is fulfilled and it is generally agreed that the concentration of potassium in the lean body mass is more variable than its water content. The concentration of potassium in the lean body mass depends on the relative amounts in different organs or tissues and the contribution that each makes to the total body weight. For example, the potassium content in the skeletal muscle in adults is between 90 and 100 meq/kg while that of the skin between 20 and 25 meq/kg but the amount varies from one muscle to another and in different parts of the skin. Most internal organs give values similar to those for muscles while the skeleton resembles the skin in this respect. Variation in the relative amounts of muscle, bone and skin will clearly lead to different concentrations of potassium in the lean body mass of different subjects, also we should expect lower concentrations of potassium in the lean body mass during infancy because, in young children, a greater proportion of the lean body mass is due to extracellular fluid than in older children and adults.

Skeletal Muscle

Skeletal muscle accounts for about 25% of the weight of newborn babies at term and about 40% of the weight of the adult male. Much of this change is due to the dramatic increase in the size of the boys' muscles which occurs during the adolescent spurt in stature.

As the muscle fibres grow, the percentage of extracellular fluid in the muscle mass falls from 67% near the end of the first trimester of gestation to 35% at term and to about 18% in the adult, but the percentages of protein and intracellular potassium increase. The muscle has not reached its mature chemical composition by the time of birth.

The age at which the muscles acquire their full number of fibres has been the subject of much discussion and the matter is still not conclusively settled. Certainly much of the growth which occurs post-natally is due to hypertrophy of existing muscle fibres. Whether or not the number of fibres increases post-natally, there is good evidence that the number of sarcolemmal nuclei increases throughout the growth of muscle. This has been confirmed histologically and also by the biochemical estimation of the amount of DNA in the muscles. The amount of DNA in a tissue can be taken as an estimate of the number of nuclei if it is assumed that all nuclei contain the same amount of DNA. In the absence of polyploidy or abnormal nuclear division, this assumption is justified for practical purposes. The increase in number of muscle nuclei is apparently due to the incorporation of nucleated satellite cells into the muscle fibre rather than the division of the nuclei already present within the fibres.

Rauh and Schumsky (1968) estimated the amount of DNA in biopsy samples of gluteal muscles. Their data suggest that the number of muscle nuclei increases throughout childhood and that the rate of increase accelerates in boys at the time of puberty so that the number nearly doubles between the ages of 10 and 16 years. During post-natal growth the number of muscle nuclei increases about 14 times. In girls the increase is smaller.

The ratio of protein to DNA provides a measure of the relationship between the amount of cytoplasm and the number of nuclei in the muscle fibres. In girls, this value becomes essentially constant after the age of 10·5 whereas in the boys it is still increasing at 16 years.

Skin

In the adult, skin represents a higher percentage (about 6%) of the total body weight than in the newborn, although the adult's surface area is smaller in relation to his body weight. This is due to increase in the thickness of the skin during post-natal growth and to a big increase in the percentage of collagen.

Bone

The matrix of the skeleton is differentiated during the first month of foetal life and bone formation begins during the second month. Most bones originate by the deposition of collagen in connective tissue, leading to the formation of cartilage in which the bone mineral is later deposited. As the cartilagenous model grows, the new cartilage on its surface quickly becomes ossified. In rapidly growing bone, calcification does not keep pace with the increase in size of the matrix and the relative amount of mineral in the whole structure falls, as for example, in the human femur during the first six months after birth. However, the ratio of calcium to phosphorus, unlike the total mineral content, remains remarkably constant during development. When growth is completed all the cartilage becomes ossified and the relationship between matrix and mineral is then more or less constant. Remodelling of the bone in later life does not appear to affect this relationship. A few bones, e.g. the clavicle and the vault of the skull, ossify directly in connective tissue or in membrane.

Before birth there is little remodelling of the cortex of long bones but this process speeds up soon after birth. During the first year of life an appreciable amount of primary bone is remodelled and secondary osteones are formed. By the end of the first year the cortex of long bones has become relatively thin, although periosteal bone continues to be actively formed, and hence the diameter of the medullary canal increases. During the second year of life, the ratio of the diameter of the cortex to that of the whole diaphysis becomes almost constant. It is probable that all the primary bone has been remodelled by the end of the second year. This implies an average rate of remodelling about ten times as great as in the adult where only some 5% of the bone appears to be remodelled each year.

Lymphatic Tissues

The lymphatic tissues, with the thymus, and the subcutaneous fat, are apparently the only exceptions to the general rule of accelerated growth at adolescence. The thymus increases in size from birth to reach a maximum at an average age of about 12 in girls and 14 in boys with a decrease occurring in the next age group. Thus the involution probably occurs at about the time of the adolescent growth spurt, but there is no exact information on this point as we only have cross-sectional data with relatively small numbers of children in each age group. Probably the lymphatic parenchyma reaches its maximum size a little earlier than is suggested by the rate of growth and involution of the whole organ. A small part of the thymus, for example, consists of connective tissue whose absolute weight continues to increase throughout puberty so that changes in the gland as a whole do not accurately reflect those in the lymphatic tissue.

The lymphatic tissue in other organs such as the spleen, intestine, appendix and mesenteric lymph nodes probably regresses at about the same time as the thymus. In the appendix the amount of lymphatic tissue is apparently greater in the 1 to 10 age group than in older subjects, while the non-lymphatic tissues of the appendix increase with age and there is some suggestion of an adolescent spurt. The amount of lymphoid tissue in the spleen increases slightly between the first and second decades but not nearly as much as other components of the organ so that there is a drop in the percentage of its total weight which is due to lymphatic tissue.

7

Interaction of Heredity and Environment in Relation to Growth

INTRODUCTION

A child's genetic make-up gives him the potential to develop specific characteristics in a predetermined sequence but he will only do so if his environment is compatible with each part of the developmental process at the appropriate time. An environment which is satisfactory at one stage of development may be unsuitable at another and therefore modify or prevent the realization of some parts of the genetic plan.

The final size and shape attained by the growing child are determined by continuous interaction between genetic and environmental forces. However, this interaction is not a simple additive one by which a given amount of "good environmental factor x" would have the same effect on everyone. For example, if all the members of a group of malnourished children were to receive an equal improvement in their diet, the resulting effect on the growth of different individuals would be very variable. The response of a child to any change in external circumstances depends not only upon his genotype but also upon the complexities of the environment which he has experienced so far. Thus, some individuals might respond excessively to a given change, while others may not respond at all and some children might react favourably to circumstances which would have an adverse effect on others.

If we wish to examine the effect on growth of any single factor in the environment, we need not only a population subjected to this factor, but also a control group which is comparable both in its genetic background and in its exposure to external conditions other than the one to be studied. For example, if we wish to observe the effect of altitude on growth, it is useless to compare a population at high altitude with a genetically and culturally different one living at a low altitude. The assumption that the two populations would react similarly to either of the two environments would not be justified without supporting evidence. There are many examples of genetically different populations reacting in contrasting ways to similar environmental conditions.

PRENATAL PERIOD

Genetic Factors

The basic plan for the development of a given region of the body appears to be established locally at an early stage of embryogenesis. For example, if a limb bud is removed from a mouse embryo and transplanted beneath the skin of an adult of the same inbred strain, it will develop bone closely resembling that of the normal adult. This implies that the basic structure of the bone is determined by the genotype and only the final modelling is the result of environmental action, namely the pressure and the pull of muscles.

A foetus may inherit genes which express themselves in abnormal intra-uterine growth. Abnormal development may also result from the presence of too many or too few chromosomes in the foetal cells and begin to manifest itself before birth. Parents who are apparently normal may transmit genes which interact to produce a pathological state in the foetus as, for example, in erythroblastosis foetalis. Certain genes may cause only slight abnormalities in heterozygous individuals but cause intra-uterine death and abortion in homozygous foetuses.

In normal intra-uterine growth, both the genotype and the environment are important. Penrose (1961) estimated that 38% of the total variation in the birthweight of a relatively large series of infants could be ascribed to heredity and 62% of the total variation was due to "environment" (24% to maternal health, 7% to parity, 1% to maternal age and 30% to unidentified factors). "Environment" in this case implies all those non-genetic influences which may act on the foetus *in utero*. Data of this kind must be interpreted with caution but strongly suggest that factors other than inheritance play an important role even during intra-uterine life. A striking example of this is provided by the length and weight at birth of monozygotic (MZ) and dizygotic (DZ) twins (Wilson, 1976). On genetic grounds alone, greater similarity would be expected in the MZ than in the DZ pairs. In fact, although the differences in size at birth are generally similar for MZ and DZ twins, the largest differences were found in the MZ group. These differences were probably due to unequal distribution of nutrients between MZ twins sharing monochorionic placentae.

Environmental Factors

The foetus may be damaged *in utero* by harmful agents acting upon it either directly or indirectly through the mother. The effect of many harmful agents is dependent upon the stage of gestation at which the foetus is exposed to them. Thus, in early pregnancy, when organogenesis is taking place, a harmful agent, e.g. a drug, may arrest the development of certain organs and result in malformation. During later foetal life, the same agent may have no effect or it might alter the overall rate of growth rather than cause malformation. Severe injury at any stage of gestation may cause foetal death, but milder injuries will not necessarily do so.

The parity of the mother, her age and the number of foetuses in the uterus influence the weight of the child at birth. First babies usually weigh slightly less than later ones irrespective of sex. Younger women tend to have lighter babies than older women although the latter are more likely to have a difficult pregnancy and delivery, with a higher incidence of congenital malformation and chromosomal abnormalities.

In a multiple pregnancy, the mother is apparently capable of supporting foetal growth without adverse effects on any one foetus until the combined foetal weight is in the region of 3·2 kg. The increase in total weight of the conceptus thereafter is essentially the same regardless of the number of foetuses in the uterus, so that the amount of subsequent growth achieved by each foetus is inversely related to the number of foetuses. The onset of labour is generally earlier in multiple pregnancies, gestation being about 237 days as compared with 281 days for single births.

It has been suggested that the interval between successive pregnancies may also have an effect on foetal growth. If pregnancies follow too closely upon each other, the mother will not have time to return to her normal physiological state between them. Attempts to determine the optimal interval between pregnancies have so far been unsuccessful.

Striking differences in mean birthweights have been reported between populations of different racial origin. Values range from 2·8 kg for

some African and Asian groups to 3·6 kg in Scandinavia. The importance of race *per se* in determining the birth weight is not clear and the
environment, particularly maternal nutrition, may be much more
important. A recent study in Guatemala showed that the babies of
mothers who received supplements of protein calories and vitamins
during pregnancy were, on average, 400 g heavier than the babies of
mothers who did not receive these supplements.

Factors such as radiation, changes in atmospheric pressure or composition and environmental temperature have been suggested as
causes of malformation and general disturbances of prenatal growth
but they may exert a greater effect after birth.

The mothers of all human foetuses are exposed to natural background
radiation which is present in varying degrees throughout the world.
Additional exposure may come from diagnostic or therapeutic procedures. Radiographic measurements of the pelvis in pregnant women
used to be undertaken quite frequently, but this technique has been
shown to be associated with higher incidence of abnormalities and a
greater risk of cancer in early childhood (McMahon, 1962). Other
authors have confirmed these findings.

In exceptional circumstances isolated groups may be exposed to
radiation as a result of industrial accident, testing of nuclear weapons,
or their use in war, as in Hiroshima and Nagasaki.

Microcephaly with mental retardation and reduced body size were
found in 10 out of 24 children whose mothers had been within 1,200 m
of the centre of the atomic explosion at Hiroshima. The incidence and
severity of microcephaly decreased with the mothers' distance from the
centre.

In another group of 30 mothers with major signs of radiation, there
were seven foetal deaths, six neonatal and infant deaths and four instances of mental retardation (Miller, 1956; Yamazaki *et al.*, 1954).

POST-NATAL PERIOD

The interaction of genetic and environmental factors continues to affect
growth and development after birth but environmental influences
become more important because the child is less well protected from
them by its mother. As the infant grows up it must adapt to an increasingly complex environment.

Genetic Factors

It is well known that children's stature is largely influenced by that of
the parents and the relationship between the two is discussed in

Chapter 3. The rate and pattern of children's growth also varies between different races. This leads to differences of adult physique which result not only from the genetic characteristics of each individual but from continuous interaction of heredity and environment. Over many generations, the growth of individuals in major populations may have been adjusted by selection so that the rate and pattern of children's development, as well as the physique of adults became adapted to the environment in which they lived. This, of course, could only happen over a long period of time and its effect on modern populations would be largely obscured by the migrations which have taken place in the last few thousand years. However, it is possible to demonstrate a negative relationship between the mean annual temperature in which populations live and their mean body weight at a given stature. Thus, members of races evolving in hot climates tend, as adults, to have a more linear build than those originating in more temperate parts of the world.

Infants descended from the African races are more advanced in several developmental characteristics than babies with European ancestry. This applies to the maturation of the skeleton in Jamaican children of African descent (Marshall et al., 1970) although the advancement is lost after the age of about three years. As economically underprivileged West Indians are more advanced than their European counterparts in better social and economic conditions, we may assume that this racial difference is genetically determined. A similar difference is found in motor development and in the eruption of the permanent teeth, although it is less obvious in the eruption of primary teeth.

After the age of about three years, underprivileged children of African descent tend to fall behind their European counterparts in rates of maturation and their growth in stature also follows a different pattern, characteristic of later maturation. This is apparently due to the economic circumstances of these children as recent surveys in the United States have shown that well-off children of predominantly African descent are taller than those of European descent. However, children of some African and Indo-Mediterranean groups are apparently shorter than Europeans when allowance has been made for social factors.

An individual's rate of maturation, as well as his size and shape is apparently determined in the genetic plan, although the environment may modify the extent to which this plan is followed. Thus, menarche which occurs at a comparable stage in the general somatic growth and development of most girls, occurs in twin sisters at ages which differ, on the average, by only two or three months. Non-identical twin sisters are, from the genetic point of view, as different as ordinary sisters but they are likely to share a common environment to a greater extent. The average difference in age at menarche of non-identical or non-twin sisters is about a year. The variation in the population at large is, of course, much wider than this. It appears that, in the West European type of population on which these observations were made, inheritance plays a large part in determining the age at menarche and probably also the age at which sexual development begins in boys.

A genetic control on the maturation of the skeleton and the eruption of the teeth apparently operates throughout childhood. Some genes do not exert an obvious effect throughout the course of development, but express themselves only in later childhood. Some are able to do so only when the body has reached a suitable state of maturation.

Developmental characteristics, such as age at menarche and final stature may be determined not by single genes but by many, each of which exerts only a small effect. We do not know how many independent genes or combinations of genes are involved in regulating the rates at which different systems approach their mature state.

Environmental Factors

Nutrition. Malnutrition may cause serious impairment of growth. The term "malnutrition" generally refers to the effects of an inadequate intake of calories, or other major dietary components, such as proteins, rather than to the specific disturbances such as rickets or scurvy which result from the lack of single essential nutrients. "Protein calorie malnutrition" is still widespread in many developing countries. Malnutrition may also result from diseases which decrease the appetite or interfere with digestion and assimilation.

Undernutrition of a relatively mild degree may inhibit growth without producing any symptoms of general disease. Prolonged or severe malnutrition, particularly in early life, may lead to kwashiorkor or marasmus. For detailed discussion of these diseases the reader is referred to standard textbooks of paediatrics.

There is abundant evidence that children suffering from malnutrition grow more slowly than those receiving an adequate diet. If the malnutrition is prolonged throughout childhood, the genetic potential for growth will not be attained and the final stature will be reduced. However, children subjected to starvation for short periods often recover more or less completely because they grow at well above the average rate when they are again given an adequate diet.

Hypoxia. People who live intermittently in high altitudes show some physiological adjustments to hypoxia but, in spite of this, their working capacity and reproductive capability may be impaired. In such groups there is a higher incidence of miscarriage, birth defect and neonatal mortality. Individuals reared at high altitude generally incur a lower risk of impairment in their reproductive or working abilities and successive generations apparently show greater cardio-respiratory adaptations. Their growth and skeletal maturation may, nevertheless, be considerably retarded as compared with populations living at sea-level (Baker, P. T., 1969). This has been observed in natives of the Peruvian Andes, who also show greater lung capacity than coastal dwellers. Whether these effects on growth are mainly due to the lack of oxygen in the environment or to other associated conditions such as cold, malnutrition and infection has not yet been established. Different races living at high altitudes in various parts of the world have apparently acquired slightly different adaptations to their environment. These variations await more detailed investigation but emphasize the importance of considering genetic and environmental factors together because the same environmental factor may interact in various ways with different genotypes.

Seasons of the year. Very few children grow at a constant rate throughout the year and most European and American data show a seasonal variation, growth being fastest in midwinter and early spring, while it is slowest at midsummer and early autumn. Growth in weight, on the other hand, is fastest in the autumn. However, detailed longitudinal studies on the changing growth rates of individual children (Marshall, 1975) have shown that only about 30% of them have cycles of increase and decrease in growth velocity which are strictly seasonal. Most of the remainder show accelerations and decelerations of growth which cannot be clearly related to the seasons. Thus if the seasons can effect growth rate, there must be other factors which are able to counteract their effect in many children. It is true however, that the growth rates of most children do vary, randomly or otherwise, in the course of the year.

Disease. Almost any illness may have some effect on growth, but acute minor illnesses, such as the childhood exanthemata or even more severe ones, such as pneumonia, do not usually cause a discernable retardation in the growth of well nourished children. There may be a greater effect in children whose diet is less adequate but this is still open to doubt. The effects on growth of chronic or repeated minor ailments are difficult to distinguish from those of other adverse factors in the type of environment with which these problems are often associated. Children with repeated colds, chronic otitis media, upper respiratory infections and skin infections are on average shorter than more healthy children. However, many of them are also subjected to sub-optimal nutrition and hygiene which may have a greater inhibiting effect on growth than their repeated minor ailments.

Serious and prolonged illnesses may cause marked inhibition of growth. The exact cause of this probably varies from one disease to another and the possibilities include reduced availability of nutrients to the growing tissues, the action of toxic substances on the growing cells, and increased production of cortisol. However severe the disease has been, its cure is usually followed by catch-up growth which in many cases is sufficient to eliminate any reducing effect on the child's final height.

Psychological Factors. Severe prolonged psychological stress can apparently inhibit growth. In a much quoted experiment, Widdowson (1951) studied the effect of increased rations on orphanage children living on a poor diet in Germany immediately after the Second World War. Her data suggested, however, that subjecting the children to emotional stress was more effective in inhibiting their growth than the increased rations were in accelerating it. More recently, the recognition of the clinical condition known as psychosocial short stature (see Chapter 9) has given further support to the view that a psychological situation which is unsatisfactory for a particular individual may cause severe inhibition of growth.

Socio-economic Class. Children of the same race but of different socio-economic status differ in average stature at all ages, the poorer children being smaller.

In the United Kingdom, the difference in height between children of the professional and managerial classes and those of unskilled labourers is about 2 cm at 3 yr but this difference increases to nearly 5 cm at adolescence. The difference in weight is less striking than that in stature because the children in the lower socio-economic groups have a greater weight for height.

The greater difference between social classes in the adolescent years is due to the earlier maturation of the better-off children. They experience the adolescent spurt while the poorer ones are still growing at a pre-adolescent rate. Even in the younger age groups, the well-off children are nearer to their final height than poor ones of the same age. Most of them are also destined to become taller adults.

The causes of this socio-economic difference in growth pattern are complicated and poorly understood. Our difficulty in understanding them is increased by the fact that, in most studies, socio-economic class has been defined in terms of the father's occupation. This is not a reliable guide to the manner in which the children are brought up.

Differences in nutrition probably play an important part in creating social class differences and are determined by the cultural as well as the economic status of the family. Both nutrition and other conditions in the home are largely dependent on the intelligence and education of the parents, especially the mother, rather than their economic circumstances, unless these are extremely poor. There is some evidence that the difference in height between parents in different social classes is maintained by a tendency for tall people to move upwards in the social scale while short people have a tendency to move downwards. There is also a lesser tendency for short daughters of skilled manual workers to marry men with skilled or non-manual jobs than is the case with taller girls of similar parentage. (Thomson, 1959).

Radiation. Radiation may affect the growth not only of children who receive excessive doses in utero but also of those who are exposed to it after birth. In 1954, a group of children were exposed to radioactive fall-out following the testing of a thermonuclear device on Bikini. The initial effects were burns, loss of hair and changes in the blood but stunting of growth and an increased incidence of thyroid abnormalities were observed later. The thyroid damage was apparently related to growth disturbance (Sutow and Conard, 1969). The effects of lower levels of radiation on human growth and development are not sufficiently well documented to permit confident interpretation.

Catch-up Growth. If a child's growth is inhibited by undernutrition, disease or lack some of the hormones necessary for growth, the effect is not necessarily permanent. If the deficiency is corrected, or the disease cured, the child will grow at a rate far above the normal for his age. As his stature approaches that which he might have been expected to reach in normal circumstances, his rate of growth slows down (Fig. 56). This phenomenon is known as catch-up growth.

The mechanism regulating catch-up growth is not known. Tanner (1963) has suggested that the central nervous system may, in some way, receive information about both the child's actual size and the size he should have reached at a given time, according to a pre-determined plan. The "mismatch" between these two signals would be a measure of the growth deficiency and would lead to an acceleration of growth in proportion to the magnitude of the deficiency. Thus the child would grow more quickly the further it was from the expected height and its growth would slow down as it approached the norm. This hypothesis, however, has not yet been tested and, in any case, it does not explain how the hypothalamus would accelerate growth on receipt of the "mismatch" signal or slow it down as the strength of the signal diminished. It is unlikely that these results would be achieved by increasing the secretion of growth hormone as exogenous growth hormone has little

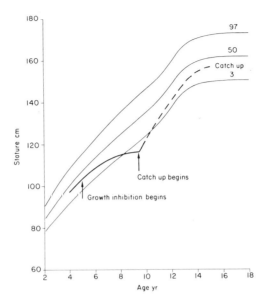

Fig. 56. Growth curve of a hypothetical child who experienced growth inhibition followed by catch-up growth.

effect on the growth of children who are not growth hormone deficient.

It is possible that a peripheral mechanism may be responsible for catch-up growth, although again, we lack evidence. However, one might envisage that a complex sequence of chemical reactions would be interrupted when growth was inhibited. Part of the sequence might continue, leading to accumulation of substrate for the later stages which could not take place. When conditions become favourable, the later reactions would proceed rapidly, owing to the large quantities of precursor available. As the supplies were used up, the rate of reaction and hence, the growth rate would slow down. The growth hormone-somatomedin mechanism might be involved.

At present, all that we can say with certainty about catch-up growth is that it almost invariably occurs when growth inhibition for a limited period after the first year of life is followed by conditions favourable to growth. We do not know why it occurs.

8

Hormones in the Regulation of Growth and Development

PREPUBERTAL GROWTH

The main hormones concerned with the regulation of post-natal growth before puberty, appear to be growth hormone and somatomedin. Thyroxine is also necessary for normal growth to occur and placental lactogen may play some part in pre-natal growth.

Growth Hormone and Somatomedin

Human growth hormone (HGH) is a protein consisting of 191 amino acids. It is species specific and although growth hormone from cattle, sheep or pigs is very similar in structure to HGH, it is not effective in man.

Growth hormone has little, if any, direct action on the growing tissues. Its effects are probably due mainly to the release of somatomedin from the liver and possibly the kidney. Hall (1971) showed that intravenous infusion of growth hormone into children who were deficient in this hormone was followed by a rise in the blood somatomedin level after about three hours, although by this time, the amount of growth hormone in the blood had fallen again to its level before infusion. The somatomedin level remained elevated for at least 24 hours. Children deficient in growth hormone have low plasma levels of somatomedin which increase when growth hormone therapy is given.

Somatomedin is believed to mediate the action of growth hormone in causing multiplication of cartilage cells and hence growth of the skeleton. However, it has yet to be demonstrated that somatomedin will cause children to grow. Also, it is not certain that growth hormone is absolutely necessary for the production of somatomedin. Some children who have undergone surgery for craniopharyngiomas are reported to have had normal serum somatomedin levels in the absence of detectable growth hormone.

Effect of Growth Hormone on Muscle and Fat

In children with isolated growth hormone deficiency, administration of HGH increases the rate of growth in width of the muscles as shown on radiographs taken under standard geometric conditions. If the treatment is discontinued the muscle width stops increasing and may actually decrease (Tanner, *et al.*, 1971).

The thickness of the subcutaneous fat, which is usually well above average in these patients, decreases during growth hormone therapy. This reflects a general decrease of body fat, in association with an increase of free fatty acids in the blood. This effect is probably mediated by somatomedin although there is no direct evidence for this.

Control of Growth Hormone Secretion

The secretion of growth hormone, like that of other pituitary hormones is apparently controlled by the central nervous system. This is suggested by the observation that a burst of growth hormone secretion occurs during early sleep and after electrical stimulation of the median eminence of the hypothalamus. However, no "growth hormone releasing hormone" has yet been isolated while a "growth hormone release inhibiting hormone" has. This substance has been characterized chemically and has been named somatostatin. The secretion of growth hormone may be regulated entirely by somatostatin or by the antagonistic action of somatostatin and a releasing factor which has yet to be identified.

The normal stimulus for the secretion of growth hormone is unknown, although many stimuli which arise in normal life, including exercise, apprehension and sleep are associated with an increase in the amount of growth hormone in the blood. Less natural stimuli, such as the ingestion of Bovril, a proprietary meat extract; the injection of arginine chloride, or the injection of insulin will also raise the blood growth hormone level in children. Apparently the output of growth hormone is not usually continuous and both children and adults produce several bursts of secretion every 24 hours.

Tanner (1972) has suggested that the normal long-term stimulus to the secretion of growth hormone may be a decrease in the blood level of somatomedin. This suggestion was based on the fact that high blood levels of growth hormone are found in children suffering from protein calorie malnutrition and with low serum protein levels. Infusion of amino acids does not lower the concentrations of growth hormone in these children and therefore the raised growth hormone level is presumably not due to a low concentration of amino acids in the serum. Also, in healthy adults, there was no increase in basal levels of growth hormone after starvation for four days or 25 days on a diet deficient in protein but with adequate calories. The difference between children and adults implies that starvation *per se* is not the essential stimulus to growth hormone secretion but that some factor in the relationship between starvation and growth was involved. As the blood level of somatomedin is now known to be reduced in starvation this might be the relevant factor.

An alternative theory is that the secretion of growth hormone is inhibited by direct action of the hormone itself on the hypothalamus. It has been shown in monkeys, whose growth serum hormone levels have been artificially raised to very high levels by intravenous infusion, that insulin hypoglycaemia will not produce any further rise. This implies that the growth hormone already in the circulation is more effective in inhibiting growth hormone release than insulin hypoglycaemia (normally a very powerful stimulus) is in stimulating it.

Abrams *et al.*, (1971) have shown that repeated injections of human growth hormone into normal young men for six days left the subjects temporarily unable to secrete growth hormone in response to insulin hypoglycaemia. The ability to secrete began to return about 12 hours after the exogenous HGH was stopped and was back to normal in about 48 hours. These results would also appear to support the hypothesis that growth hormone itself is an essential agent in the feedback control of growth hormone production. However, Tanner (1972) suggested that the time relationship in this experiment would be in keeping with the view that somatomedin is the essential feedback agent.

ENDOCRINOLOGY OF PUBERTY

The somatic changes which take place at puberty vary greatly not only in the age at which they occur but also in their relationship to other measures of maturity such as skeletal age. Furthermore, they do not occur in the same order in all children. It is therefore clearly wrong to regard puberty as a single process. The endocrine phenomena associated with breast development, genital development, pubic hair growth, the adolescent growth spurt and other events must be considered independently of each other. Unfortunately, this concept is overlooked in much of the endocrine literature, where puberty is usually discussed as if it were a single sequence of events.

Our knowledge of the complex hormonal changes underlying puberty is still very limited. The testes, ovaries, adrenals, and thyroid show a rapid increase in weight at puberty. The anterior pituitary also has a spurt of growth which is greater in girls than in boys. Before puberty there is very little, if any, difference between the sexes in either weight of the pituitary or the volume of the sella turcica. The bigger pituitary in girls after puberty is due to a greater increase in the number of acidophil cells, possibly those that secrete prolactin. However the size of the gland, or even its hormone content, is not a good measure of the amount of hormone which it is manufacturing or secreting.

Reliable methods for estimating the amount of various hormones in the blood and urine are a recent development and the estimation of secretion rates is still largely impossible. Some hormones, such as growth hormone and luteinizing hormone, are secreted only intermittently in response to either some inherent cycle or an external stimulus. Because of this, we should have to take continuous blood samples for the whole 24 hours in order to obtain integrated secretion rates, and information about normal children is therefore practically non-existent. Also, as in the study of most aspects of development, we are more concerned with changes over a period of time rather than with the state of the individual at a given moment. In other words, we need longitudinal studies. Unfortunately, very few longitudinal studies of endocrine events during adolescence have been carried out.

Care is also necessary in interpreting biochemical assays of hormones in the blood or other fluids as these techniques do not necessarily measure the amount of biological activity which is present. For example, the standard method of estimating pituitary hormones, radioimmunoassay, measures only a short sequence of five or six amino acids in a molecule which may consist of one or two hundred. We cannot be certain that the sequence which we are measuring is the one with biological activity.

Ideally, chemical assays should be validated against bioassays, but this is not always technically possible. Chemical assays, once validated have the great advantage that they are much less laborious and are often more reliable and more sensitive. Also they are usually more specific. These provisos must be borne in mind in the following discussion.

Gonadotrophins

Both FSH and LH can be detected in the blood by radioimmunoassay from birth onwards. They are also present in the urine. Earlier bioassays were not sufficiently sensitive to detect the small amounts present in early life, or to distinguish between FSH and LH, but this is now possible. Cross-sectional data suggest that, in boys, the concentration of either substance in the blood does not change appreciably from early childhood up to the age of 6. Between 6 and 10 yr there is a gradual, but significant, rise in the mean levels of both. Boys whose ages varied between 9·6 and 15·1 yr, but who showed signs of early puberty (i.e. testicular enlargement) had significantly higher FSH and LH levels than prepubertal subjects. When the mean values of FSH in boys aged from 10 to 17 were plotted against age, regardless of the subject's state of sexual development, the curve continued to rise but the slope was not significantly greater than in younger children and several 10-year-olds showed values within the adult range. On the other hand, the curve of serum LH values did increase in slope after the age of 12.

In girls, serum LH values remained low and there was no significant increase until after sexual development had begun. FSH levels were high in some infants and the values decreased with age to reach a minimum at eight years, followed by a rise coincident with puberty. After menarche, high levels of both FSH and LH were found in some subjects but the range of variation was very wide, presumably as a reflection of the gonadotrophin surge in mid-cycle (Faiman and Winter, 1974).

The same authors carried out a mixed longitudinal study in which blood was taken once a year for four years from 56 normal boys aged from 6 to 14 and once a year for three years from 58 girls aged from 6 to 16 at the beginning of the study. The age range was thereby covered by a series of short-term longitudinal studies. Special statistical procedures were used to produce estimates of the mean changes, which were unbiased by the subjects entering or leaving the study. Figure 57 shows the mean values of FSH and LH and testosterone plotted against chronological age while Fig. 58 shows the hormone levels in each stage of puberty. Unfortunately, the puberty stages were assigned by combining genital and pubic hair stages and not by separate criteria for each

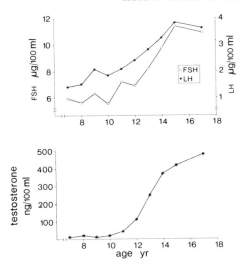

Fig. 57. Serum levels of LH, FSH and testosterone in boys at different ages. The data are semi-longitudinal. (Redrawn from Faiman and Winter, 1974).

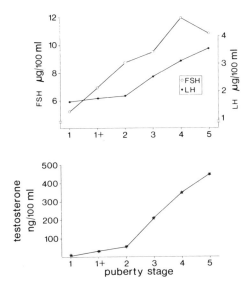

Fig. 58. Serum levels of LH, FSH and testosterone in boys at different stages of puberty. Stage 1+ refers to subjects who advanced to stage 2 in the following year. (Redrawn from Faiman and Winter, 1974.)

character. Figure 58 shows that FSH rises first, increasing by just under 50% from stages 1 to 2 while neither LH nor testosterone change significantly. FSH continues to rise and reaches the adult male value shortly before development of the genitalia and pubic hair is complete. LH, on the other hand, begins to rise only after stage 2 and continues to do so up to stage 5. The curve for testosterone is similar. More restricted cross-sectional data by other authors are in agreement with these results.

In girls, Faiman and Winter (1974) found a pattern of increase of FSH and LH similar to that in the boys. Figure 59 shows the mixed

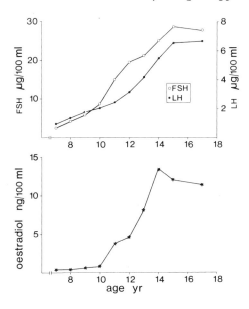

Fig. 59. Serum concentrations of LH, FSH and oestradiol in girls at different ages. (Redrawn from Faiman and Winter, 1974.)

longitudinal data plotted against chronological age. Both FSH and LH increased gradually in the 7 to 10 age group and at age 10, FSH began to rise more steeply than LH.

Finkelstein *et al.* (1973) recorded plasma LH levels every 20 minutes throughout 24 hours in a number of children and adolescents. When LH first began to rise it did so in bursts during sleep. Later the bursts also occurred during wakefulness but the sleep bursts remained predominant, giving a mean value of 13·3 miu/ml during sleep as compared with 9·6 miu/ml whilst awake. When puberty was completed, the sleep and waking values became equal.

The urinary output of gonadotrophins may be better than isolated blood samples as a measure of the 24 hour production rate, because the hormones are probably released intermittently. An increased rate of production might be achieved either by releasing more at each burst or by increasing the frequency of pulses of hormone release. We can measure only the amount of hormone present in a blood sample at the time it was taken but we may expect the blood level to fluctuate in relation to the pulses of hormone release, and therefore to be a poor measure of the total production of hormone. A 24 hour sample of urine gives us a measure of total hormone output, provided the amount of hormone in the urine is proportional to that of the blood. The output of gonadotrophin in 24 hour collections has been studied by a number of investigators, but only the results of cross-sectional studies have been published so far.

FSH concentrations rise in the urine during early puberty just as they do in the blood, and reach maximal levels by stage 3 or 4 in boys (Raiti *et al.*, 1969; Baghdassarian *et al.*, 1970). Urinary LH, on the other hand, showed a considerable increase after stage 4 had been reached, although there was also a rise in early puberty. Quantitatively, the LH excretion in adulthood is about 12 times greater than in childhood, whereas FSH is only four times greater. Amongst boys at any given stage of puberty, there is a wide variation in the amount of gonadotrophin which can be detected in either blood or urine.

Gonadal Hormones

Testosterone. The concentration of testosterone in boys' blood falls during the first week of life but rises again to reach a new maximum at 1 to 3 months, which is similar to the levels found in puberty. However, this high concentration is not maintained and has fallen to a very low level by about the seventh month. In girls the level at birth is lower than in boys and falls in the first week. There is no subsequent rise in the first year. This sex difference in testosterone production in the neonatal period may influence later development of the hypothalamus or reproductive organs, although as yet, there is no evidence as to its precise significance.

The urinary excretion of testosterone increases gradually in the years before puberty and appears to be similar in the two sexes up to the age of about 11. After this, the boys show a much greater increase than the girls. Mean values for adult men are nearly ten times as great as those for pre-adolescent boys while women secrete only about three times as much as pre-adolescent girls.

The longitudinal data of Faiman and Winter (1974) (Figs 57 and 58), indicate that plasma testosterone levels in boys rise only slightly until the secondary sex characters begin to develop and then very steeply until stage 5, when mean values of between 13·88 nmol/l and 17·36 nmol/l are reported. The rise continues beyond this point, however, and mean levels of 20·83 to 24·31 nmol/l are found in young adult men. The final stages of hair growth may be dependent upon these higher levels of testosterone as the moustache and beard are not usually fully grown and the axillary hair may be incompletely developed until some time after stage 5 has been reached.

Plasma testosterone apparently rises in girls as well as in boys, although to a lesser extent. In pre-pubertal girls, Faiman and Winter (1974) found mean levels similar to those in pre-pubertal boys, i.e. about 0·7 nmol/l. The value in girls rose to about 1·38 nmol/l in early puberty, with stage 2 or 3 pubic hair and to 1·74 nmol/l in post-menarcheal girls. This level of testosterone is found in boys about stage 2, i.e. when they have much less pubic hair than most adult women, and is presumably insufficient to sustain the adult growth of pubic hair in males. However, post-menarcheal girls have been exposed to slightly raised levels of testosterone for a much longer time than boys in early puberty. It is conceivable that a testosterone level of 1·38 or 1·74 nmol/l might cause boys to have hair growth similar to that of the adult female if they were exposed to it for a sufficiently long period. On the other hand, the skin of females may be more sensitive than males to testosterone and other circulating androgens. Testosterone in women is believed to come largely from the peripheral conversion of androstenedione secreted by the ovary and adrenal (Horton and Tait, 1966).

An important event in the action of androgens is the 5α-reduction of testosterone to dihydrotestosterone which is further metabolized in the target cells leading to the production of androstanediol (5α-androstane-3α-17β-diol). The rate of this last conversion is higher in men than in women (Mahoudeau *et al.*, 1971) and the amount of androstanediol which can be detected in the boy's plasma increases about 13 times during the course of sexual development.

The ratio of androstanediol to testosterone increases in early puberty, but, by the time sexual maturity is reached, it has declined again to approximately its prepubertal level (Gupta, 1975). The ratio of dihydrotestosterone to testosterone follows a similar pattern. The initial rise in these ratios suggests that there is an increase of 5α-reductase activity in the tissues during early puberty.

Oestrogen. The oestradiol level in the blood of both sexes is higher at birth than it is during most of childhood. The levels fall rapidly within a few hours and then decline more gradually. During the second week of life, in girls, the plasma oestradiol rises again to levels similar to those found during puberty. They remain high for about a month and then fall but do not reach normal prepubertal levels until about the sixth month. The rise in boys is probably less than that in girls.

Oestradiol levels rise again in girls as the changes of puberty advance and adult levels are reached by the time of menarche or soon after (Faiman and Winter, 1974). However, there is wide variation between individuals at all stages of sexual development and even from day to day in the same subjects. The urinary excretion of oestrone, oestradiol and oestriol increases with sexual maturation.

In boys, plasma oestradiol rises in early puberty to its adult level which is similar to that of girls in breast stages 2 or 3. The source of oestradiol in the male is not known.

Plasma oestrone levels are similar in boys and girls at comparable stages of sexual development. Oestrone, which in girls is believed to come mainly from the adrenal and not the ovary, has the same range of values as oestradiol in both sexes from age 1 to 6. However, from ages 7 to 10 the mean value for oestrone increases before there is any similar rise in oestradiol (Saez and Morera, 1973). This suggests that the adrenal may increase its production of oestrone before puberty.

Adrenal Androgens

There is a dramatic increase in androgen secretion by the adrenal at adolescence. Adrenal androgens may be largely responsible for the adolescent growth spurt in girls and the adrenal cortex is the main source of androgens in adult women. In men, adrenal androgens are of little importance as compared with testosterone, but they do provide precursor steroids in the synthesis of testosterone. They may also provide substrate in the synthesis of oestrogens.

In Blood. The principal androgens found in blood from the adrenal veins of both men and women are dehydroepiandrosterone and its sulphate; 11β-hydroxyandrostenedione and smaller quantities of androstenedione. In mixed venous blood, however, dehydroepiandrosterone sulphate and androsterone sulphate are the most prominent substances, but very little of either is detected in the mixed blood of children under the age of about 7. After this, the quantity appears to increase steadily and, just before puberty, is equal to about one-third of the amount found in young adults. A sharp rise may occur at puberty but confirmation of this would require longtitudinal data which are not yet available.

In Urine. As in the case of the gonadotrophic hormones, it can be argued that the urinary output during 24 hours of androgens and their metabolites gives a truer picture of adrenal hormone production than we can obtain from isolated blood samples.

The 17-oxosteroids in urine may be divided into two subgroups.

i) The 11-oxy-17-oxosteroids include further metabolites of androstene-dione and metabolites of cortisol. They are not a useful index of androgen production and will be discussed no further.

ii) The 11 deoxy-17-oxosteroids, derived from dehydroepiandrosterone (DHA) and androstenedione (Fig. 60). DHA itself is found in the urine together with aetiocholanelone and androsterone which are derived from androstenedione. The output of these substances in 24 hour samples of urine is a reasonably accurate reflection of adrenal androgen secretion in boys and girls before puberty and in adult women but, in adult men, testosterone also contributes.

The urinary output of all three 11-deoxy-17-oxosteroids increases from about 7 years of age with a more dramatic rise at about 11 years, which continues until about the 18th year. The increase in DHA is less than that of aetiocholanelone while androsterone, which has greater androgenic properties than aetiocholanolone, shows the greatest increase. The steep rise in total 11-deoxy-17-oxosteroids which occurs in the urine at about the time of puberty is still apparent when the results of the assays are expressed in relation to height, weight or surface area. It is therefore not merely an adjustment to increasing body size.

Longitudinal studies of a small number of children (Gupta and Marshall, 1971) showed that the urinary output of androsterone was, in fact, increasing slowly from the 3rd birthday (when the study began) and a more rapid increase began at ages 5 and 6 in some individuals (Fig. 61). In another longitudinal study beginning at age 8, Tanner and Gupta (1968) found that androsterone began to increase dramatic-ally at ages which varied between 8 and 11 in different subjects (Fig. 62). Their skeletal ages at the beginning of this rise varied between 9·5 and 11·5.

There is very little sex difference in DHA secretion before the age of 11 but, at 14, the upper limit of the range of variation for girls is approximately equal to the lower limit of the range for boys. Boys excrete more androsterone than girls from about the age of 12.

The Cause of Increased Androgen Production. We do not know why adrenal androgen output increases before puberty. It is unlikely that the rise is due to ACTH as the production of corticosteroids does not increase at the same time. It is also unlikely that LH is responsible because the LH content of the blood and urine does not increase until after the secondary sex characters have begun to develop. Also premat-ure adrenarche (i.e. the early development of the pubic hair without breast development in girls) is not associated with a rise in LH while

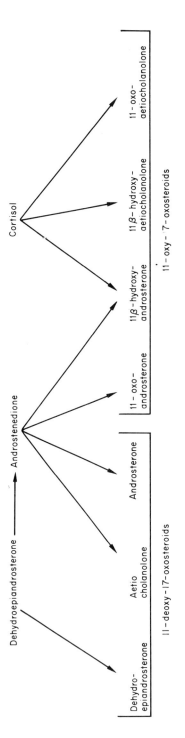

Fig. 60. Derivation of individual 17-oxosteroids. (Redrawn from Forsyth, 1974.)

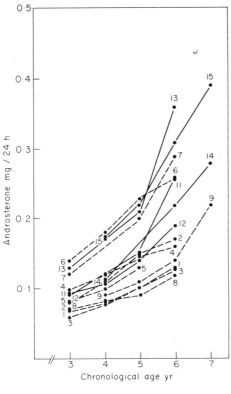

Fig. 61. Urinary output of androsterone in a number of children
studied longitudinally by Gupta
and Marshall (1971). With permission.

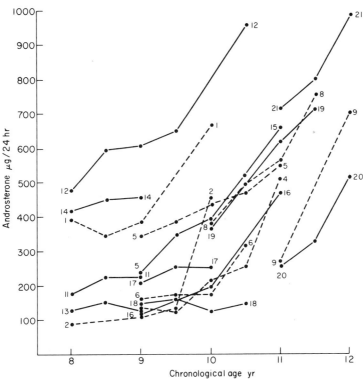

Fig. 62. Urinary output of androsterone in a number of children studied longitudinally by
Tanner and Gupta (1968). With permission.

increased blood levels of LH in certain other conditions, including castration and administration of gonadotrophins to adult eunuchs, are not accompanied by an increased output of adrenal androgens. There is no direct evidence that FSH influences the adrenal.

On the other hand, the injection of human chorionic gonadotrophin is said to increase the plasma level of DHA in pre-pubertal children. However, this need not imply a direct action of gonadotrophin on the adrenal and is in keeping with the alternative view that steroids of gonadal origin, either androgens or oestrogens, stimulate the production of androgens by the adrenal. Experiments *in vitro* suggest that androgens and oestrogens inhibit 3β-hydroxy-dehydrogenase enzyme activity in the adrenal, in such a way that the metabolic pathway leading to the formation of corticosteroids is slowed down to a greater extent than the pathway leading to the production of androgens. Also administration of testosterone to prepubertal boys leads to an increased output of both 11-deoxy-17-oxosteroids and 11-oxy-17-oxosteroids but does not cause a rise in cortisol metabolites.

Occasionally congenital adrenal hyperplasia presents at puberty when the cortisol deficiency, which was previously mild, becomes pronounced. This too might be explained by the action of androgen or oestrogen in the adrenals. The fact that cortisol deficiency does not develop at puberty in healthy children may be due to increased production of ACTH.

Gonadotrophic and gonadal hormones may act synergistically to stimulate adrenal androgen production at puberty. However, longitudinal studies, in which all the relevant hormones and metabolites are assayed repeatedly in the same subjects before, during and after puberty, are necessary to clarify the situation.

The Initiation of Puberty

Puberty may occur in an essentially normal way, but at a very early age, in children with certain brain lesions and sometimes quite young children reach full reproductive capacity. For example, the youngest mother on record gave birth to a healthy infant by caesarian section at the age of 5 years 8 months. Also, development of the breasts and penis may occur in small children who have ingested sex hormones. Clearly, therefore, the secondary sex organs are sensitive to stimulation by androgen or oestrogen at a much earlier age than that at which puberty normally occurs, and it is unlikely that change in this sensitivity plays an important part in the initiation of puberty. Hence we must assume that the mechanism is a central one.

If the pituitary of a newborn rat is grafted beneath the hypothalamus of an adult rat, it soon begins to release hormones just like a normal adult pituitary. This indicates that it is the maturity of the central nervous system and not of the pituitary itself which determines whether gonadotrophins should be released in pre- or post-adolescent amounts. The central nervous system exerts its influence through the medium of gonadotrophin releasing hormone (GnRH).

Small amounts of sex hormone are circulating in the blood of young children and there is evidence that these inhibit the output of gonadotrophins, presumably by inhibiting the output of GnRH. On the basis of animal experiments which have recently received some support from clinical data (Grumbach *et al.*, 1974), it has been suggested that, at puberty, the hypothalamic cells, which regulate the production of gonadotrophins, become less sensitive to the inhibitory action of androgens and oestrogens.

As a result, the small amounts of these hormones in the circulation which, until this change occurred, were sufficient to inhibit the production of GnRH, now fail to do so. The level of sex hormone in the blood therefore rises until it is again sufficient to inhibit gonadotrophin production at a new higher level. The feedback circuit is thereby re-established with circulating levels of gonadotrophin and sex hormone which are sufficient to initiate and maintain the development of the secondary sex characters.

As puberty advances, a "positive feedback" apparently develops in the female so that rising blood levels of oestrogen cause increased secretion of LH from the pituitary. This "LH surge" plays an important part in the mechanism of ovulation.

There is some evidence that, in addition to the above "re-setting" of the feedback mechanism, the gonadotrophin producing cells of the pituitary may become more sensitive to GnRH as puberty approaches. This would lead to a greater output of gonadotrophin in response to a given amount of GnRH. This in turn may reflect the accumulation of increasing reserves of FSH and LH in the pituitary.

Regulation of the Adolescent Growth Spurt

Adrenal androgens, in girls, with the addition of testosterone in boys, are known to be important in accelerating growth at adolescence. However, recent studies by Tanner and others of growth hormone deficient children have shown that growth hormone is also necessary to produce a spurt of normal magnitude. Apparently testosterone acts almost entirely on the growth of the trunk while growth hormone is essential for the growth of the limbs. About one-third of the total gain in stature during adolescence may be dependent upon growth hormone.

9

Short Stature: Differential Diagnosis and Treatment

INTRODUCTION

When parents complain that their child is too small or is growing very slowly their complaint must be treated seriously even if the child appears to be in perfectly good health. If they say that his growth was previously normal but has recently slowed down, this may be the first indication of a serious disorder, even though the child's present stature is within normal limits. Inhibition of growth due to disease, particularly of the renal or alimentary systems, or an intracranial lesion, may persist for some time before the symptoms of the underlying condition are sufficient to cause either the child or his parents to complain. Growth failure may also reveal endocrine disorders which are amenable to treatment or psychological and social problems which can be relieved if appropriate advice and help are made available. Even when short stature is not due to any underlying abnormality it can be a major source of worry to a child and his parents. We can help these children considerably by giving reassurance, after adequate investigation, and indicating what the child's growth prospects are likely to be.

Parents may have various reasons for thinking that their children are "not growing properly" but some of the commonest modes of presentation are as follows:

i) the child is not gaining weight at the rate which they expect;

ii) he is not growing out of his clothes as quickly as he used to, or not at all; he is the smallest in his class at school; (this is commonly noted either at the beginning of the child's school career or from the age of about 11 onwards, in a child who is not experiencing the adolescent growth spurt at the same age as many of his peers. At this stage also, a late maturing boy may be alarmed by the discovery that he is smaller than many girls of his own age.)

iii) a younger brother or sister may become taller than the patient;

iv) the parents may themselves be small and hope that steps may be taken to prevent their child being equally small as an adult.

In all these circumstances there are two conditions which require our attention. One is the parents' and/or the child's anxiety, which may be considerable. The other is the child's supposedly abnormal growth. Before we can deal with either of these problems we must ascertain whether or not the patient's growth is in fact abnormal, using the methods described in Chapter 3. After this we can either offer reassurance or proceed with further diagnostic procedures and, in some cases, with successful treatment.

SHORT STATURE ASSOCIATED WITH GROSSLY ABNORMAL APPEARANCE

Some children with short stature look essentially normal apart from their size but others show striking abnormality of the shape or proportions of the trunk and limbs. The latter group includes those who have abnormally short limbs as in achondroplasia, hypochondroplasia and various rare bone disorders. Abnormalities of the face are also found in many rare conditions such as the Cornelia de Lange syndrome or the mucopolysaccharidoses. The webbed neck, widely spaced nipples and wide carrying angle are well known characteristics of Turner's syndrome but the chromosomal disorders associated with these stigmata may be present in children whose appearance deviates very little, if at all, from the normal range of variation. Most of the conditions in which short stature is accompanied by an abnormal overall appearance are too rare to merit discussions in this book. The most important ones are mentioned briefly but, for more detailed information the reader is referred to the excellent books by Smith (1970) and Bailey (1973).

Achondroplasia

Achondroplasia is characterized by short limbs. This shortening is particularly noticeable in the upper arm and thigh where there are often rolls of soft tissue and transverse skin creases. The hands and feet are short and broad. The fingers are approximately equal in length and cannot be fully adducted. This results in the "trident hand" typical of this condition. The patients are muscular in appearance and the head appears large with a prominent forehead and chin. The nasal bridge is depressed. There is marked lumbar lordosis and a protuberant abdomen. Radiographs of the skull show brachycephaly and increased vertical diameter with a small foramen magnum. In the absence of this last finding the diagnosis of achondroplasia is suspect. The twelfth thoracic or first lumbar vertebra is often hypoplastic and posterior concavity of the vertebrae is characteristic of this condition. The vertebral canal narrows from above downwards. The long bones of the limbs are, of course, short. The femur has a short neck with prominent greater and lesser trochanters. The fibula is less affected than the tibia and is therefore relatively long.

There are no abnormal biochemical findings and there is no effective treatment, although secondary effects such as impaired circulation of the cerebrospinal fluid and ear infection may call for intervention.

Genetic counselling may be required. Achondroplasia is inherited as an autosomal dominant condition but mutation accounts for about 85% of the new cases seen. The abnormal gene may be transmitted by either parent to children of either sex. If a heterozygous achondro-plasiac were to mate with an unaffected person, 50% of their children would, in theory, be affected.

If two heterozygous achondroplasiacs were to mate, 25% of their children would be homozygous for the condition; 50% would be hetero-zygous, but equally affected, while 25% would be normal and would not transmit the condition to their own offspring. If a normal couple produce an achondroplasiac child, their chances of having another affected child are no greater than for any other normal parents. If they did have another, the diagnosis should be reconsidered as there would be a greater likelihood that an autosomal recessive condition was being transmitted.

Hypochondroplasia

Shortening of the limbs is less marked than in achondroplasia. The face and skull are essentially normal, both clinically and radiographically. The hands, although small, are of normal shape, in clear distinction to the "trident" hands found in achondroplasiacs. Narrowing of the inter-peduncular spaces of the vertebrae is less marked in hypochondroplasia than in achondroplasia.

Although both these disorders exhibit an autosomal dominant mode of inheritance, they are believed to be quite independent of each other. This implies that a hypochondroplasiac is no more likely than an unaffected person to produce an achondroplasiac child. The offspring from the mating of an achondroplasiac with a hypochondroplasiac may show either condition but no intermediate forms have been reported.

Severe cases of hypochondroplasia may be difficult to distinguish from mild achondroplasia. Mild cases of the former condition may also be difficult to recognize.

Diastrophic Dwarfism

Diastrophic dwarfism is also characterized by short limbs but the forearms and lower legs are affected to a greater degree than the upper arms and thighs. There is marked talipes equinovarus with limitation of movement at other points leading amongst other things to a characteristic "hitch-hiker thumb" deformity. Soft swelling occurs in the external ears. Cleft palate is found in about 25% of cases.

Further deformities develop with increasing age and the management of these is the main aspect of treatment. The mode of inheritance appears to be autosomal recessive.

Metaphyseal Dysostosis

This term refers to a group of disorders characterized by deficient ossification of the metaphyses. Radiographs show splayed irregular metaphyses with radiotranslucent areas which give an appearance suggestive of rickets. The defects are not always confined to the limbs and the spine may be affected to varying degrees. At least fifteen different types of metaphyseal dysostosis have been described but the most common is that known as the Schmid type. Affected patients are moderately short in stature. They have tibial bowing, especially at the ankle; waddling gait with coxa vara; flared lower rib cage and limited extension of the fingers. Radiographs also show broad, irregular, splayed metaphyses. The Schmid type shows an autosomal dominant mode of inheritance, but many of the other types are autosomal recessive.

Mucopolysaccharidoses

This is a group of six conditions characterized by increased urinary excretion of mucopolysaccharides, with short stature and other abnormalities. The intelligence is usually severely impaired, except in the case of mucopolysaccharidosis IV (Morquio's syndrome) where it is usually normal. The best known mucopolysaccharidosis is Hurler's syndrome in which signs of physical and mental deterioration follow normal development in early life. The cranium becomes disproportionately large; the nostrils are wide and the nasal bridge depressed; the tongue is enlarged and thick and hypertelorism is common. The limbs and trunk are also deformed and the abdomen is protruberant. Diagnosis is confirmed by analyses of mucopolysaccharides in the urine. The disorder is inherited as an autosomal recessive trait and treatment is purely symptomatic.

Cornelia de Lange Syndrome

In this syndrome the eyebrows meet, the eyelashes are long. The upper lip is narrow, tending to curve downwards, and is described as "carp like." The fingers and toes are short. Growth is impaired before birth. The intelligence is low. There is no laboratory test by which the diagnosis can be confirmed.

Prader–Willi Syndrome

Patients with this syndrome are typically short and obese. Hypogonadism and cryptorchidism are found in affected boys. The eyes are usually almond-shaped with hypertelorism, epicanthus and strabismus. The ears are low-set and the mouth shows a high arched palate, enamel hypoplasia and micrognathia. The hands and feet are small. A characteristic feature of this syndrome is hypotonia in the neonatal period. Sucking and swallowing are usually poor. Muscle tone usually improves after a few months but developmental milestones such as sitting and walking are usually delayed.

Obesity usually begins by the age of two years and increases throughout childhood. Excessive deposition of fat is most obvious on the trunk, buttocks and proximal parts of the limbs. In older children, the intelligence varies from severely subnormal to normal. Diabetes mellitus may appear in later childhood.

The aetiology of the syndrome is unknown, although a hypothalamic disturbance has been suggested.

SHORT STATURE WITH ESSENTIALLY NORMAL GENERAL APPEARANCE

Variations of Normal Growth

Some small children are essentially normal and their short stature is inherited from their parents. The method of deciding whether or not a child's stature may be regarded as normal, when his parents' stature is taken into consideration, has been discussed in Chapter 3. There is at present no treatment which will cause the normal child with inherited short stature to reach a greater height than that determined by his genotype.

Some children are small for their age during childhood only because they are late maturers and are not so near to their final stature as most other children of the same age. They usually experience puberty rather late and are therefore still growing at a pre-adolescent speed while their classmates at school are experiencing the adolescent growth spurt. The smallness of these children in relation to their peers becomes increasingly noticeable from the age of about 11 in boys and a little earlier in girls and this is the age at which they most commonly seek medical advice. The bone age is usually considerably less than the chronological age. The terms "slow maturation" or "slow tempo of growth" as suggested by Tanner (1973a) are most appropriate to describe these children. Some authors have used the term "delayed puberty" as a diagnosis, even when the patients are well below the age at which puberty normally occurs. However, it is clearly ridiculous to say that a 5-year-old is suffering from delayed puberty. The growth curve of a typical child with slow maturation is shown in Fig. 63.

There is no satisfactory treatment for slow maturation during childhood. Sex hormones may be given to the teenager who is very concerned about his or her lack of sexual development but, in general, this is undesirable. Administration of androgens to a boy causes his secondary sex characters to develop but the testes remain small. Skeletal growth is accelerated and the immediate results of treatment therefore seem satisfactory but, unless great care is taken with the dosage of androgens, the bone age may increase very quickly. As a result of this, the patient's growth may stop before he has reached the stature which he would have attained if the treatment had not been given. Occasionally, the combined effects of relatively late puberty and short stature creates psychological problems serious enough to outweigh the disadvantages of androgen therapy. In these cases, androgen may be given but the skeletal age should be checked at least every six months so that the dosage can be reduced, or the treatment stopped, if it appears that the final stature is likely to be below acceptable limits. The acceleration of skeletal maturation caused by androgen treatment may not be apparent for the first six months and then there may be a dramatic acceleration which outweighs the gain in height. Because of these risks, the use of androgens to treat children suffering from slow maturation

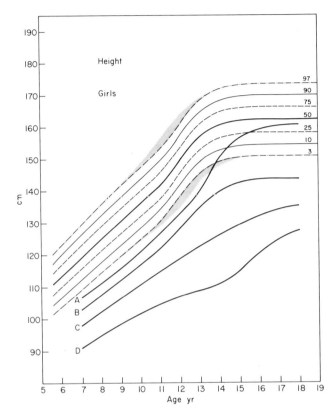

Fig. 63. Growth Curves typical of various categories of small children: A = normal child with slow maturation; B = child who had low birthweight for her gestational age; C = Turner's syndrome; D = growth hormone deficiency (untreated).

should be carried out only under the supervision of a specialist.

If either oestrogens or androgens are given continuously over a period, fertility may be jeopardized. Gonadotrophins are often given as an alternative treatment but it is doubtful if there is any real advantage in this. Androgens should never be given to genetically short children whose bone age and sexual maturation are not delayed. This would almost certainly reduce their potential adult height. In fact, we shall see in the next chapter; oestrogens and androgens may be used to reduce the final stature of girls and boys who are too tall.

Short Stature in Various Diseases

Almost any disease in childhood may cause growth to slow down or stop.

However, recovery is usually associated with a period of accelerated or "catch-up" growth, in which the child grows at a greater than average rate until he reaches approximately the stature he would have achieved if the illness had not occurred. The growth rate then returns to normal (see Chapter 7). It is difficult to assess how much effect a short-term illness has on stature because it is almost immediately corrected by catch-up growth. A prolonged illness which retards the growth rate may reduce the final stature, depending on the extent to which skeletal maturation is also impaired. If the development of the bones is retarded by an amount equivalent to the deficiency of growth in height, then catch-up growth may occur without any diminution of the final stature. On the other hand, if skeletal maturation continues more or less normally while growth in height has slowed down or stopped, then the ultimate height will be reduced, unless catch-up growth occurs without correspondingly accelerated increase in bone age.

The diseases which are major causes of short stature are considered here only in relation to their effects on growth. For further details of diagnosis and treatment, the reader is referred to standard paediatric texts.

Nutritional Disorders. Malnutrition resulting from an insufficient intake of food is a well-known cause of short stature which is still regrettably common in the world at large. It is, however, rare in the developed countries and is a special topic beyond the scope of this book. However, malnutrition may occur *in utero* and in the neonatal period even when adequate supplies of food are available. Therefore, in all cases of short stature careful note must be made of the patient's birth weight, the mother's health during the pregnancy and any other available information about growth and nutrition during the neonatal period. Malabsorption of protein, fat and carbohydrates, either collectively or individually, may cause malnutrition of sufficient severity to inhibit growth, although the underlying cause may not be clinically obvious.

Carbohydrate malabsorption usually presents as a severe, acute illness following gastroenteritis or other intestinal disease and is a problem for the emergency admission team rather than the clinic which deals with growth disorders. However, primary deficiencies of intestinal disaccharidases occasionally present as failure to grow. The patients usually have watery stools.

Fat malabsorption (steatorrhoea) is more common than defective carbohydrate absorption. Normally, absorption of fat takes place largely in the upper small bowel, after the fat has been emulsified by pancreatic juices and bile salts and hydrolized by intestinal pancreatic lipases to glycerides and fatty acids. Steatorrhoea may result from impairment of either the emulsification and hydrolysis process or from impaired absorption.

When fat malabsorption is due to biliary obstruction, growth failure is usually only part of a clinical picture which does not create a difficult diagnostic problem. In disorders of the pancreas, as in cystic fibrosis, short stature may be the only presenting symptom. As effective replacement therapy is available in cases of pancreatic deficiency, it is important that these patients are correctly diagnosed.

The malabsorption associated with Crohn's disease is probably due to intestinal hurry, as normal absorption can occur only if the food remains in contact with a competent bowel surface for an adequate length of time. However, malabsorption may not be the major cause of growth failure in this disorder as some patients have shown no evidence of steatorrhoea and yet their growth has been seriously impaired. The reason for this is unknown.

Coeliac disease may seriously impair growth and must be diagnosed because it responds well to treatment. The main feature of this disease is an abnormality of the villi of the mucosa of the small bowel. This results in great reduction of the effective absorptive surface of the bowel. When gluten is excluded from the diet, the villi reappear and there is a marked improvement in general health and in growth. Some children with coeliac disease have no intestinal symptoms and the only apparent abnormality is short stature which may be associated with low skinfold thicknesses. The diagnosis can be established with certainty only by demonstrating the characteristic mucosal abnormalities on jejunal biopsy. Indeed, because coeliac disease responds so well to treatment there is a good case for suggesting that a jejunal biopsy should be carried out on all children with short stature whose cause cannot be diagnosed otherwise.

Obstruction to the lymphatic drainage from the bowel occurs in intestinal lymphangiectasia where it is due to abnormality of the lacteals, and in some other conditions. As a result, dietary fats cannot be absorbed and steatorrhoea develops. In addition, lymph may be exuded into the bowel causing hypoproteinaemia which, in addition to the effects of fat malabsorption, increases the severity of the effective undernutrition.

Chronic gastrointestinal infection may lead to malabsorption and is common in many parts of the world. It is less frequent in developed countries with temperate climates, but chronic giardiasis sometimes occurs, especially in institutions. Colonization of the bowel by abnormal flora may follow surgery, when the bowel contents may become stagnant, usually as the result of adhesions.

Protein malabsorption may accompany fat malabsorption, whenever this occurs, but especially in diseases of the pancreas. However, loss of protein into the bowel is more important than protein malabsorption as a cause of severe protein malnutrition. Protein losing enteropathy may occur whenever the bowel is injured, as in coeliac disease, and protein loss may be the major defect in diseases which affect the lymphatics of the bowel wall. This may be the reason why growth impairment is more marked in these conditions than in other malabsorptive states.

Renal Disease. Renal disease is an important cause of growth failure and should always be considered in the differential diagnosis. The most common renal disorder in childhood is urinary tract infection. This has been found in many completely asymptomatic children, most of whom are not excessively short but might have been taller in the absence of the infection. However, relatively mild symptoms of chronic or recurrent urinary infection are sometimes associated with quite severe impairment of growth and, if the infection is eliminated, catch-up growth will usually occur. When untreated urinary tract infection is allowed to progress to chronic pyelonephritis and renal failure, growth is severely impaired.

Renal tubular disorders are rare but they cause serious failure in growth which is presumably due to the loss of phosphate, hydrogen and potassium ions, together with amino acids and water. The diagnosis of these disorders is a highly specialized subject.

Cardiovascular Disorders. Growth impairment is common in congenital heart disease and is probably due to low oxygen saturation of the tissues. A right-to-left shunt causes deoxygenated blood to pass into the systemic circulation while a large left-to-right shunt may recirculate oxygenated blood to the lungs and thereby reduce the effective cardiac output. When short stature is due to congenital heart disease, the primary cause is usually obvious.

Respiratory Disorders. Chronic respiratory insufficiency (most commonly asthma) may result in slow growth. However, one cannot emphasize too strongly the warning that asthmatic children may suffer much greater impairment of growth as a result of a long-term treatment with corticosteroids than would be caused by the asthma itself. These substances should be used only if there is no satisfactory alternative therapy and, even then, the dosage should be kept as low as possible. Anoxia is not essential for respiratory disease to impair growth; for example children with widespread bronchiectasis usually have subnormal growth rates even when their arterial oxygen saturation is apparently normal. In these cases the growth failure is probably due to the chronic infection rather than damage to the respiratory system *per se*. Chronic infection of any organ may have this effect although some children with severe infection grow quite normally.

Disorders of the Blood. Chronic anaemia is usually associated with growth failure. The commonest cause is a congenital haemolytic anaemia (e.g. thalassaemia major) but other acquired anaemias, e.g. iron deficiency anaemias, have the same effect. In tropical and sub-tropical regions hookworm infestation, together with an inadequate diet, is one of the major causes of anaemia. There should be little difficulty in diagnosing anaemia which is sufficiently severe to cause growth failure as other symptoms, due to anaemia itself, will attract more immediate attention than the child's lack of growth. If therapeutic measures are successful in preventing prolonged severe anaemia, normal growth may occur. For example, when thalassaemic children are given blood transfusions, their growth velocities may return to normal although catch-up growth frequently does not occur. The patients therefore do not make up the growth which they lost as a result of their disease prior to treatment and remain small. Puberty is usually greatly delayed.

Liver Disorders. Obstructive jaundice impairs fat absorption by restricting the supply of bile salts. When the condition is of long standing it will therefore result in short stature even if secondary liver damage is minimal or absent. In chronic liver diseases the synthesis of protein is impaired and this is probably the main cause of growth failure which accompanies these disorders.

Cerebral Disorders. Many children of very low intelligence have short stature, but there is no simple relationship between stature and intelligence as such. Sometimes there is a common cause for both the short stature and the low intelligence, as for example, in children whose birth weights are low in relation to their gestational ages ("small for dates" babies). Many of these children are small but some are of normal or high intelligence while, in others, the intelligence is impaired, presumably as a result of the same intra-uterine factors that impaired their somatic growth *in utero*.

Biochemical Disorders. Abnormal calcium metabolism may cause serious impairment of growth. Hyperparathyroidism is rare in childhood but hypercalcaemia due to excessive administration of vitamin D was not uncommon in the recent past. This was usually the result of giving vitamin D supplements in addition to powdered milks, which were themselves fortified with vitamin D. Now that the risk of failure to thrive as a result of this practice is widely recognized, the condition is becoming less common.

Idiopathic hypercalcaemia is a rare cause of short stature but, if it is not treated, the child's intellectual development may be greatly impaired and the kidneys may suffer permanent damage. Hence it is important that this condition should be diagnosed but it is not easy to recognise clinically. The serum calcium should therefore be checked in any baby who fails to thrive. The condition is believed to be due to increased sensitivity to vitamin D.

Hypocalcaemia is not difficult to diagnose clinically if tetany occurs but this is seldom seen in children and the diagnosis usually depends on biochemical evidence. Neonatal hypocalcaemia is usually transient and in later childhood the condition is due to rickets, renal disease or parathyroid disorders. Dietary rickets had become uncommon in most highly developed countries but is again being found more frequently, especially in immigrant populations from Asia, and has persisted in the indigenous populations of some regions. Rickets is common in countries where the standard of living is very low. When the diet is adequate, rickets may result from malabsorption or from renal disease. Short stature may be the only presenting symptom.

Primary hypoparathyroidism is rare but pseudohypoparathyroidism (characterized by hypocalcaemia and hyperphosphataemia) and pseudopseudohypoparathyroidism (in which the plasma calcium and phosphate levels are normal) are now being diagnosed more frequently and may not be as rare as was formerly thought. In both these conditions (which are variants of a single pathological condition known as Albright's Hereditary Osteodystrophy) short stature, sometimes quite severe, is usually the presenting symptom. In addition, there are abnormalities of the metacarpals and metatarsals, ectopic calcification and rather low intelligence. There may not be any other associated biochemical abnormalities. It has been suggested that the underlying cause is a peripheral block to the action of parathyroid hormone which is present in unusually high amounts. If the serum calcium is low, vitamin D and additional calcium may raise it but this does nothing to repair the underlying defects nor does it produce any noticeable improvement in growth.

Many of the rarer inborn errors of metabolism, which are beyond the scope of this book, may also be associated with growth failure.

Absent or Abnormal X-Chromosome

When the second sex chromosome is absent, giving karyotype 45XO, the result is Turner's syndrome. The patient's stature is usually well below the 3rd centile and up to the age of about 9 or 10 the growth velocity usually remains just within normal limits, i.e. at about the 10th centile on the velocity chart. The centile status of the patient on the stature chart therefore drops gradually. At about the age of 11 or 12, when we should expect the adolescent growth spurt to occur, it does not do so. Instead, growth slows down gradually for a few years before it finally stops (Fig. 63.) In childhood the skeletal age is usually close to the chronological age, or a little below it, but after the age of 12 or 13, the skeletal age falls progressively behind the chronological age.

The diagnosis can often be made on clinical grounds although it should be confirmed by cytogenetics. At birth, there may be lymph-oedema with characteristic residual puffiness over the dorsum of the fingers and toes. Other stigmata present at this time, often become more obvious as the child gets older. The chest is broad with widely spaced nipples, which may be hypoplastic, inverted or both. The auricles are often unusually prominent and the neck is short, sometimes with a "web" of skin extending laterally to the shoulders. The hair line is low. Variable abnormalities of the skin, skeleton, cardiovascular and renal systems may also be found. The germinal elements of the ovary are hypoplastic or absent in 90% of cases and therefore the breasts do not develop at puberty, and menstruation is either absent or very scanty and transient. Pubic hair is usually sparse and sometimes does not appear. A small mandible and inner canthal folds give a characteristic facial appearance to some patients.

Clearly, girls with the complete form of Turner's syndrome are not entirely normal in appearance but patients with chromosomal mosaicism, i.e. one line of cells with the 45XO karyotype, and another with a normal 46XX karyotype (or perhaps a different chromosomal abnormality) are often entirely normal in appearance although they may exhibit the characteristic stigmata to some extent. In some, the growth pattern is similar to that of children with pure 45XO karyotypes and the breasts do not develop; others have some adolescent spurt and varying degrees of breast development. In the most fortunate, growth and breast development may be essentially normal.

The diagnosis of chromosomal abnormality must be considered in all girls with unexplained short stature, as there need not be any other stigmata. Absence of sex chromatin in the cells of the buccal mucosa is a useful indication of a 45XO karyotype but, in mosaic patients, the buccal mucosa may be normal in this respect. A complete cytogenetic study is therefore necessary to exclude the diagnosis and should be done as a routine on every girl with short stature who has not been otherwise diagnosed.

There is no treatment for the underlying disorder but oestrogens may be given to produce breast development. The dosage should be kept to the minimum which will achieve the desired result in each patient. There is some evidence that androgens in small dosage may have a beneficial effect on growth but this matter requires further study before the treatment can be recommended.

A phenotype similar to that of girls with Turner's syndrome, but occurring in boys, is known as Noonan's syndrome. However, no chromosomal abnormality has been demonstrated in these cases.

Unsatisfactory Environment

In utero—"Small for Dates" babies. An unsatisfactory intra-uterine environment may adversely affect a child's growth both before and after birth although, of course, slow growth *in utero* may also be due to factors inherent in the zygote or foetus itself. Slow intra-uterine growth results in a low weight at birth, even if gestation continues for forty weeks. If the gestation period is less than this, the weight of the newborn baby will be low in comparison with that of healthy babies born at the same gestational age. When the gestational age (or, strictly speaking, the post-menstrual age) is known, the "small for dates" babies can easily be identified with the aid of charts which give centiles for birth-weight at different gestational ages, e.g. those produced by Tanner and Thomson (1970) (Figs 17 and 18). These children frequently suffer from short stature in later life. It is important that they should be distinguished from infants who are born before term but whose rate of growth *in utero* was normal. These children do not usually show any abnormality in their post-natal growth and are called "preterm with normal weight." "Preterm" is defined by international agreement as less than 37 weeks gestation.

If the gestational age is not accurately known, one has to decide the approximate length of gestation on the basis of observations made at birth, frequently by another medical practitioner or by a midwife, and measurements made during pregnancy, using clinical or ultrasound techniques will also be helpful if they are available. It is important to realize, however, that the various clinical techniques which are designed to measure gestational age do not, in fact, do so. They measure only certain aspects of the child's maturity and compare it with that of the average child of a given gestational age. This makes no allowance for normal variation. Healthy infants who have survived *in utero* for any given number of weeks may be at different levels of maturity, just as normal healthy 10-year-old boys may have bone ages which vary between 8 and 12 "years." At birth, however, the "maturational age" of the baby may be more important than its true gestational age. A discussion of the various techniques used to estimate foetal maturity would be inappropriate here. If a child is unusually small, it is important to know whether or not his size at birth was appropriate for his gestational age but this information can be obtained only from the case history as the patients do not usually present themselves with this problem until several years after birth.

When the newborn infant is abnormally small in relation to its gestational age there may be some recognizable pathological or genetic abnormality. In most cases, however, the cause is not immediately obvious and a diagnosis such as "foetal malnutrition", "placental insufficiency" or "chronic foetal distress" is often given without any clear justification. These babies often exhibit soft tissue wasting, which suggests that malnutrition frequently accompanies intra-uterine growth retardation.

In some cases an apparent cause of foetal growth inhibition can be found, e.g. severe toxaemia of pregnancy, single umbilical artery, twinning, severe maternal starvation or massive placental infarction. Usually, however, the cause is not obvious although there is a statistical association between low birth weight and cigarette smoking in mothers; low maternal weight before pregnancy or a history of growth retardation in younger sibs. Socio-economic and racial factors are less important but the incidence is increased in primipara and grand multipara.

Some "small for dates" babies may recover from their intra-uterine growth inhibition by growing quickly after birth. However, many grow only at about the average rate from birth onwards and do not recover from the set-back which they suffered *in utero*. They therefore remain small throughout childhood and become small adults (Fig. 63).

As "small for dates" babies grow into childhood, they often develop a characteristic appearance: they are usually rather thin, the mandible is small in relation to the maxilla, the corners of the mouth are turned downwards and the ears appear low set in relation to the face.

The fifth fingers are usually short and curved inwards and sometimes the limbs, trunk or face show a degree of asymmetry which is beyond normal limits. The condition without asymmetry has been known as "Russell syndrome" while it has been called "Silver's syndrome" if asymmetry is present. However there is no valid ground for this distinction and, if an eponym must be used, Silver–Russell is most appropriate (Tanner *et al.*, 1975).

When a child is at, or below the 3rd centile and growing at a normal rate, the diagnosis of intra-uterine growth retardation should always be considered although, in the case of a girl, Turner's syndrome or one of its variants is equally possible in the light of this evidence alone. There is, as yet, no treatment which will effectively increase the final stature of children with intra-uterine growth retardation.

After Birth. Undernutrition and chronic or recurrent infection are the most common environmental factors which inhibit post-natal growth. Undernutrition of sufficient severity to inhibit growth, in the absence of disease, is rare in most developed countries. Where it does occur it is essentially a social problem and education of the mother, so that she gives her children a proper diet by using the resources available to her, is often more important than providing the economic means to obtain more food, although this may also be necessary. Education in matters of hygiene is the most important step towards minimizing those infections which are associated with poor social conditions.

"Psycho-social" short stature has now been recognized as a clinical entity. The patients may come from families where the other children are growing normally but the patient himself grows at a subnormal rate while he remains at home. His growth rate improves considerably if he is moved from his home to another environment and demonstration of this is the only means of confirming the diagnosis. There is some evidence that the secretion of growth hormone is impaired in these patients while they are at home and that their improved growth elsewhere is associated with increased ability to secrete growth hormone. Catch-up growth can be quite dramatic and similar to that of growth hormone deficient children who are treated with growth hormone.

Endocrine Disorders

The major endocrine causes of short stature may be considered under four headings as follows.

Iatrogenic. An important cause of short stature is the administration of cortisone and related substances to children suffering from asthma, skin disorders and other diseases. Quite small doses will inhibit growth of some children while other patients will tolerate larger amounts and grow more or less normally. It is therefore impossible to suggest any particular dosage which is safe for general use. The long-term use of steroids in treatment of children should be avoided wherever possible but, when their use is essential, the dosage should be kept to the minimum which is compatible with the child's well-being. It is not entirely clear whether ACTH therapy is less inhibitory to growth than the use of corticosteroids as there is some conflict in the evidence currently available.

Growth Hormone Deficiency. Children who lack the ability to secrete growth hormone are usually extremely small in comparison with others of the same age. Their birth weights are usually normal but their growth rates are usually below average from birth onwards. In later childhood the growth rate is nearly always below the 10th centile, and usually below the 3rd when it is plotted on the velocity charts. The patient's stature therefore falls progressively below the 3rd centile. The growth curve of a typical untreated patient is compared in Fig. 63 with those of children with other growth disorders. The skeletal age is usually considerably less than the chronological age and the stature may therefore fall well within the normal range if it is plotted against bone age. Apart from their small size, the appearance of these children is essentially normal but they tend to be rather fatter than average and the boys often have small genitalia. Their intelligence is usually quite normal.

The differential diagnosis includes delayed maturation in a normal child; psycho-social short stature; chromosome abnormalities (especially XO/XX mosaicism where the general appearance may be normal) and hypothyroidism. Occasionally children with malabsorption or renal disease are sufficiently small and normal looking to be included in this differential diagnosis but the former are usually thin.

The diagnosis of growth hormone deficiency can usually be confirmed by radioimmunoassay of the serum growth hormone before and after a suitable stimulus such as exercise, Bovril (a proprietary meat extract which temporarily raises the serum growth hormone level in normal children) or intravenous insulin. Usually one of the first two stimuli is used as a general screening procedure, while intravenous insulin is used to confirm the result when the first test shows an abnormally low level of growth hormone. The insulin test should only be carried out by an experienced physician, with all the precautions necessary to control the level of hypoglycaemia. Isolated estimations of serum growth hormone without a prior stimulus are of little value as the blood level varies greatly in normal children, and may be very low indeed on some occasions.

Children whose short stature is due to psycho-social problems may show a poor growth hormone response to one of these stimuli if it is given whilst the child is living at home. A normal response will usually be found if the test is carried out after the child has been removed from his home and kept in hospital for a few days or weeks.

Growth hormone deficiency may occur in isolation or it may be accompanied by a deficiency of other pituitary hormones. Deficiency of ACTH or TSH can be recognized by the appropriate clinical tests. A deficiency of gonadotrophins cannot at present usually be diagnosed until the age at which puberty would be expected to occur.

In all cases of growth hormone deficiency it is essential to exclude the possibility that a craniopharyngioma or other tumour may be the cause of the defect. Growth hormone deficiency, in the absence of a tumour, is much commoner in boys than in girls. Conversely, the incidence of tumours is much higher in growth hormone deficient girls than in boys. No adequate explanation has yet been offered for this sex difference.

There is a tendency for more than one case of growth hormone deficiency to occur within some families, but a family history occurs in only some 3 to 5% of cases. There is some association between growth hormone deficiency and breech birth. There is also some association with forceps delivery in multipara. There is good evidence that some patients may suffer from a partial deficiency of growth hormone and these may be difficult to distinguish from those with simple delay of maturation.

Patients with growth hormone deficiency can now be successfully treated with preparations of human growth hormone. The response to therapy is often dramatic, as shown in Fig. 64, but a few patients have developed antibodies to the hormone, with the result that it has become ineffective. No other adverse side effects have been reported. In the United Kingdom this hormone is available within the framework of a trial organized by the Medical Research Council. Some other countries have similar arrangements for its distribution. At present, the hormone can only be obtained by extraction from the pituitaries of human cadavers.

When growth hormone deficiency develops during later childhood or adolescence, some serious underlying pathology is likely to be present. The clinical picture is usually one of a previously normal child whose growth rate is steadily falling. This situation can only be recognized by the correct use of stature and velocity charts. Once the growth failure has been recognized it constitutes an alarm signal for thorough investigation. There are many diseases which could result in this clinical picture but growth hormone lack due to craniopharyngioma or other CNS lesions is one of the most likely.

Hypothyroidism. The short stature and typical appearance of the severely hypothyroid child is well known and is not difficult to recognize. Real myxoedoma is seldom seen in young children but puffiness round the eyes and localized subcutaneous pads in the supraclavicular regions are characteristic. The head often seems large and the neck appears very short. The hair may be coarse and dull in appearance while the hair line is low-set, especially in front of the ears. The tongue often tends to protrude, enhancing the suggestion of low intelligence which is confirmed by appropriate testing.

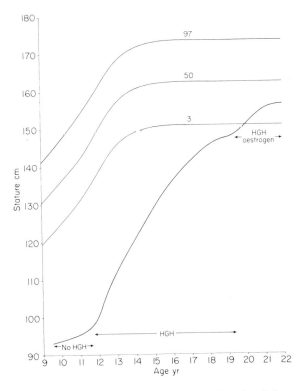

Fig. 64. Growth curve of a patient with hypopituitarism, treated wtih human growth hormone and, later, with human growth hormone plus oestrogen. Data kindly supplied by J. M. Tanner.

However, some children with mild hypothyroidism may be essentially normal in both appearance and intelligence but have subnormal growth rates and delayed skeletal maturation. Short stature is the presenting symptom in these patients who are clinically not dissimilar to those who lack growth hormone. However, the diagnosis is established by appropriate tests of thyroid function. The serum growth hormone does not usually rise in response to Bovril or to insulin-induced hypoglycaemia but does so when the patient is treated with thyroxine. Treatment with thyroxine usually causes a dramatic acceleration of growth in the patients, until they eventually reach a final height as great as, or perhaps even greater than, they would have reached in the absence of hypothyroidism. Great care is required in adjusting the dosage of thyroxine as the blood level must be sufficient to accelerate growth without causing disproportionate advance in bone age. If the maturation of the skeleton is accelerated too much the ultimate stature will be reduced.

Disorders of the Pituitary Adrenal Axis. Congenital adrenal hyperplasia, in its commonest form, is accompanied by sexual precocity and acceleration of both somatic growth and skeletal maturation. The patients are therefore tall as children but their growth stops at a very early age and they become relatively short as teenagers and adults.

Relatively short stature in later childhood is a feature of many children with precocious puberty (see Chapter 4) whatever its cause. In some cases the final stature may be below the 3rd centile although the patients are tall in early childhood.

Cushing's syndrome, with its characteristic obesity, "moon face" and striae is usually suspected from the patient's appearance. However, in children, short stature rather than obesity may be the presenting complaint. The child may also experience back pain, muscular weakness and hirsutism. Evidence of virilization is not uncommon, with acne, penile enlargement or clitorial hypertrophy, and scrotal pigmentation. In adolescent girls, secondary amenorrhoea is frequent.

10

Tall Children: Differential Diagnosis and Treatment

MODE OF PRESENTATION

Sometimes tall parents who have found their tallness to be an embarrassment or handicap, are afraid that their children will become as tall or even taller than they are themselves. These children are often brought for assessment at a very early age, when their stature or supine length may be well within normal limits and no prediction as to their future growth prospects can be made.

Other parents are concerned because their son or daughter is taller than many acquaintances of the same age. A few children are sufficiently tall to be brought to medical attention for this reason while they are still pre-adolescent, or even in infancy. However, this problem is much more common between the ages of 9 and 13, usually in girls. Those who experience the changes of puberty, and hence the adolescent growth spurt, at a relatively early age become much taller than their peers who are still pre-adolescent. They are embarrassed by the immediate situation and are also afraid that they will become abnormally tall women.

Usually the only presenting symptom is tallness, although in some adolescent girls the main concern may be "big feet". This problem arises because the feet usually reach their adult size before the rest of the body, whilst further increase in stature is yet to come. The feet appear disproportionately large at this time, but the child's fear that they will continue to grow and become enormous, is rarely justified.

ASSESSMENT

The first object in assessing a tall child is to make sure that the tallness is not due to any underlying pathology. If a condition amenable to treatment (e.g. pituitary adenoma) is recognized, the tallness *per se* becomes a secondary consideration. The underlying disorders must be fully assessed and the appropriate treatment arranged. If no abnormality is found, the next steps are to predict the patient's final stature and decide whether or not treatment aimed at reducing the final height is appropriate.

In taking the history, particular attention should be paid to the child's earlier growth, attainment of paediatric milestones and performance at school. Any history of ophthalmic or cardio-vascular disorder in either the patient or the family should be carefully noted. The statures of the parents, and as many other relatives as possible, should be recorded together with the statures of the siblings. In the case of an adolescent girl it is important to ask whether or not menstruation has begun and if so, when. The clinical examination should include measurement of stature and sitting height as described in Chapter 1, and the development of the secondary sex characters should be noted in accordance with the stages described in Chapter 4. A record should be made of any unusual features such as linearity of body build, a narrow palate, unusual facial features or abnormalities of the hands and feet. The hands may be disproportionately large or they may be unusually long in relation to their breadth. An X-ray of the left hand and wrist, suitable for estimation of bone age, should be taken.

The child's stature is plotted on a centile chart. In the majority of patients who seek medical advice because of their tallness, the stature is not grossly abnormal and it is often within the normal range of variation, i.e. close to the 97th centile. However, a stature at, or even below, the 97th centile does not exclude those disorders of which tallness is a feature. Neither does it establish that the patient will not eventually become so tall as to have considerable social disadvantages.

If we plot the parents' statures on the same chart as their daughter's we can make at least an approximate judgement as to whether the child's growth is typical of the family. If a tall child has rather short parents, the tallness is more likely to have a pathological origin than in the tall child of tall parents. An adjustment to the parents' height has to be made before it can be plotted on the chart of the child of opposite sex. Five inches (12·7 cm) is added to the mother's height before she is plotted on her son's chart. Similarly, 12·7 cm is subtracted from the father's height before he is plotted on his daughter's chart. This correction allows the parent of the opposite sex to the patient to be plotted on the correct centile.

If the child is between 2 and 9 years of age, we can make a more exact appreciation of the normality of his stature in relation to that of his parents by using the charts of Tanner *et al.* (1970). These charts, which are described more fully in Chapter 3, show the distribution of heights in normal children after allowance has been made for the stature of their parents.

TALLNESS OF PATHOLOGICAL ORIGIN

Excessive Growth Hormone Production

This is mentioned first because, thanks to generations of undergraduate textbooks, it is the most well known. In fact, it is exceedingly rare in childhood. It is doubtful whether it always leads to excessive growth and it may or may not be accompanied by signs of acromegaly before growth in stature has stopped. It usually leads to acromegaly later. A pituitary adenoma of sufficient size to produce neurological symptoms is seldom found in children or adolescents but there may be one which can be detected radiographically. Enlargement of the pituitary fossa may be seen on routine skull radiographs and the paranasal sinuses may also be enlarged. The hand and wrist X-rays taken for the prediction of the final height should also be examined for the "tufting" of the phalanges which is suggestive of acromegaly. If there is any suspicion of a pituitary adenoma, further investigation by specialized radiological techniques will usually be required to define the exact position and size of the tumour.

In adult acromegalics, the concentration of growth hormone detected in the blood by radioimmunoassay is often abnormally high and in some patients this concentration is not reduced by increasing the blood glucose levels, as it is in most normal subjects. The serum insulin concentration is also raised in acromegalics. Estimations of serum-growth hormone and insulin during a glucose tolerance test are therefore useful in the assessment of acromegaly. Similar tests are of some value in studying tall children and adolescents but their use is at present limited by a lack of comparative data in tall normal children. It may be incorrect to interpret children's results in the same way as those obtained when the test is carried out in adults.

In those rare cases where evidence of a pituitary adenoma is found, the tumour may be ablated by surgical or radiotherapeutic methods. If the other circumstances of the case permit, it may sometimes be preferable to postpone this treatment until the changes of puberty are completed unless, of course, damage caused by the tumour is already so extensive that puberty will not occur.

Cerebral Gigantism (Soto's Syndrome)

Children with this condition are big at birth and grow very quickly in the first three or four years but their final height may not be excessive. The patients have a characteristic facial appearance due to a rather long skull, usually with frontal bossing, and eyes which are rather far apart with an antimongoloid slant. The chin is elongated with thick subcutaneous tissues which give the lips a thickened appearance. Radiographs of the skull show enlarged frontal sinuses but the sella turcica, although usually large, is within normal limits. The skeletal age is usually advanced in relation to the chronological age. Occasional nonspecific EEG abnormalities have been reported.

The serum growth hormone level is normal and the intelligence may be normal but is usually low. This, together with the child's very large size, and often poor coordination, makes social adjustment in childhood very difficult. There is no satisfactory treatment other than general support for the parents. The administration of androgens or oestrogens, which may reduce the height attained by normal children, is of little value in this situation, where the main problem is excessive size in childhood and not in adult life. In the case of boys, androgens would cause a spurt of growth which would make the situation worse during treatment. Only in those few cases where it is obvious that the adult height will be excessive should hormonal treatment be considered.

Marfan's Syndrome

Patients with this disorder are usually rather tall, although their final stature is seldom above the normal range.

The main features of the syndrome are long slim limbs, with particularly narrow hands and long fingers (arachnodactyly). There is little subcutaneous fat. The joints show hyperextensibility and, associated with this, there may be scoliosis and kyphosis. In the eye, subluxation of the lens, with defect in the suspensory ligament and retinal detachment may be found. The intelligence is normal.

The ascending aorta may be dilated, with or without dissecting aneurism. Less commonly the thoracic or abdominal aorta or the pulmonary artery is dilated and there may be secondary aortic regurgition. Serious vascular complications may develop at any age and are the chief cause of death. The mean age of survival is about 43 years for men and 46 years for women. The syndrome is hereditary and therefore the family history plays an important part in the diagnosis.

The final stature of patients with Marfan's syndrome is seldom great enough to justify treatment with hormones to limit their growth. Furthermore, the possibility that androgen and oestrogen therapy might adversely affect the ophthalmic and vascular complications of the syndrome must be borne in mind.

Homocystinuria

This disorder may be difficult to distinguish from Marfan's syndrome. The patients are rather tall with a slim build. They may also have arachnodactyly, subluxation of the lens and medial degeneration of the aorta and elastic arteries. However, patients with homocystinuria are usually of subnormal intelligence and the diagnosis can be established by a chemical estimation of homocystine in the urine. No completely satisfactory treatment is available yet. As with Marfan's syndrome, the final stature is rarely enough to justify any attempt to limit growth. In girls, the administration of oestrogen for this purpose is positively contra-indicated as it might precipitate thrombo-embolic phenomena which are the most dangerous feature of this disorder.

Other Rare Causes of Tallness

Hyperthyroidism is a rare cause of tallness which should be considered in the differential diagnosis. In Berardinelli's Lipodystrophy syndrome there is accelerated growth and hyperlipaemia in early childhood. Hyperglycaemia may develop later. The hands, feet, penis and liver are enlarged while the muscles are hypertrophied and there is a lack of adipose tissue from early life. Death may result from cirrhosis of the liver with oesophageal varices. The Wiedemann–Beckwith syndrome consists of macroglossia, omphalocoele, macrosomia and cytomegaly of the foetal adrenal. Early post-natal growth may be rather slow but later stature is usually in the region of the 90th centile and skeletal maturation has advanced. Prognosis beyond childhood is unknown at present.

Precocious puberty causes tallness in childhood although it is associated with advanced skeletal maturation which leads to an early cessation of growth. As a result of this, the patients may become unusually short adults. The precocious sexual development is, however, obvious, and its possible causes are discussed in Chapter 4. The treatment is that of the underlying cause.

Patients with the syndrome of testicular feminization are sometimes unusually tall (see Chapter 4).

NORMAL TALL CHILDREN

Most children who seek medical advice because of their tallness do not suffer from any of the above disorders, and are perfectly healthy. Our task then is to decide whether or not the patient's final stature will be so great as to constitute a serious handicap. We have to distinguish between the tall child who is destined to become a tall adult and the one who is simply an early maturer, whose growth will stop before the stature has become excessive. Having done this, we are in a position to discuss with both child and parents whether any treatment should be given.

Interpretation of Height Prediction

The method of predicting adult height is discussed in Chapter 5, where the range of error in children of different ages is also given. It is not possible to make predictions as accurately as we would like for clinical purposes. Also we must remember that both the prediction technique itself and the estimates of its errors, are based on the study of children whose statures varied within the normal range. Very few of them were unusually tall. The accuracy of both the Bayley and Pinneau and the TW2 method when applied to healthy girls whose statures are already above the 97th centile requires further investigation. However, the work of Roche and Wettenhall (1969) suggests that the Bayley and Pinneau method probably has about the same accuracy in tall girls as in others and this is probably true of the TW2 method (Zachmann *et al.*, 1975). Neither method is valid when applied to girls whose tallness is of pathological origin. A height prediction allows us to distinguish with reasonable certainty between those girls who are going to be very tall e.g. in the region of 6 ft 3 in (190 cm) or more and those whose final stature will be quite acceptable. Clearly we should consider any available treatment for the former group while the latter should not be treated at all. However, in practice, most patients fall between these two extremes and it is difficult to decide whether or not treatment should be offered.

Consider, for example, a healthy 10 year-old girl whose predicted adult height is 5 ft 11 in (180 cm). The possible error of this prediction is such that she might reach 6 ft 1 in (185 cm) but may stop growing when she is only 5 ft 9 in (175 cm). By repeating the prediction two or three times, at intervals of a few months, we might be able to make a subjective judgement as to whether the first prediction was too high or too low, but the outcome would still be uncertain.

If we could offer a treatment which was absolutely safe and could be guaranteed to reduce the final stature by a predetermined amount, there would be little difficulty in reaching a decision in collaboration with both the child and parents as to whether it should be used. The only available medical treatment, however, is unpredictable in its effects on both the growth and general well-being of the patient, while most parents, and many surgeons, are unwilling to consider shortening the legs surgically.

Treatment – Girls

Medical. Tall girls may be treated with oestrogen. The most satisfactory regime is probably ethinyl oestradiol in a dosage of 0·3 mg daily with norethisterone 10 mg daily for the last four or five days of every four weeks. It is advisable to begin with 0·1 mg daily of ethinyl oestradiol and increase the dosage gradually to 0·3 mg if there are no immediate side-effects (e.g. nausea, oedema or hypertension). Some authors favour other preparations and the best for one patient may not suit another. The principal alternatives are stilboestrol, which sometimes causes unsightly enlargement and pigmentation of the areola, and conjugated oestrogens which have the disadvantage that they contain substances of unknown effect. Oestradiol valerate has the disadvantage that it must be given by injection and, because of its prolonged action, cannot be discontinued immediately if side effects develop. It may, however, be useful for girls who suffer from nausea when taking oral oestrogen.

Mean reductions in final height (as compared with predictions before treatment) of between 3·5 and 4·5 cm have been reported by several authors. However, the reduction in individual girls has varied from about 10 cm to a negative value (i.e. the patient finished up slightly taller than the predicted height). Thus we cannot forecast how effective the treatment will be and in some cases it may have no effect at all.

It appears that, in addition to increasing the rate of skeletal maturation, oestrogens may actually reduce the rate of growth in stature but their exact mode of action is not clear. There is evidence that they do not reduce the blood level of growth hormone and may even increase it. However, some authors have reported that the output of somatomedin is suppressed by oestrogen. This could explain the reduction of growth velocity in girls receiving oestrogen therapy, but does not account for the acceleration of their skeletal maturation. Zachmann *et al.* (1975) have suggested that large doses of oestrogen, as used in the treatment of tall girls, may increase the output of androgens and thereby indirectly accelerate the maturation of the skeleton.

The possible dangers of oestrogen therapy must not be overlooked. The association between oral contraceptives and thrombo-embolism is well-known, but the author is not aware of any serious instances of this in girls being treated with oestrogen to reduce their stature.

Wettenhall, *et al.* (1975) reported mild thrombosis of the superficial veins of the calf in one girl out of the total number of 168 whom they have treated with stilboestrol. In this case there was a family history of intravenous thrombosis. Hypertension and liver damage are other possible side effects which have not been observed in practice. It has not yet been fully established that oestrogen therapy does not impair the fertility of some patients in later life. Some girls have become pregnant after treatment and delivered healthy babies, but most of those who have been treated are not yet married. We cannot therefore assume that the treatment is free from risk although in the short term the danger appears slight. There may be long-term effects which we have no reason to suspect at present.

The possible dangers should be discussed fully with the parents and oestrogen should not be prescribed unless they are fully convinced that the risks are outweighed by the threat to their child's happiness created by her potential stature. The parents should also be warned that the treatment is not always effective and that we cannot predict its effectiveness as far as their child is concerned. In the author's opinion, oestrogen therapy is seldom justified unless there is a reasonable possibility that the child's final stature will exceed 6 ft (183 cm).

Oestrogen therapy causes almost immediate development of the breasts and vaginal bleeding usually occurs after the first few months. The treatment should therefore not begin until these changes would be acceptable to the patient without causing psychological or social difficulties. This is usually about the age of 10 but clearly depends on the age at which sexual maturation begins in her peers. It is probably advizable to begin as soon after this as possible although there is now some evidence that the treatment may be effective even if it does not begin until after menarche has occurred naturally. Unfortunately it is difficult to make an exact judgement on this point as we can only estimate effectiveness by comparing the patient's true final height with her predicted height. It is quite possible that the true final height would have been less than the predicted value in some cases even if oestrogen had not been given.

Surgical. Surgical shortening of the lower limbs has the advantage that it need not be carried out until the patient's growth is completed. He or she then knows the true final stature and has discovered whether or not it is creating social problems which justify this treatment. The amount by which the limbs should be shortened can be decided in advance and, as many tall women have relatively long legs, the operation need not make them disproportionately short. The risks of this type of surgical procedure are well known and can be fully discussed with the patient. Some orthopaedic surgeons are unwilling to undertake this form of treatment while others regard it quite favourably.

Treatment – Boys

Medical. In boys, tallness is not so great a social handicap as in girls and there are very few in whom the need for treatment is sufficient to outweigh the disadvantages.

Boys may be treated with androgen, which is usually given by injection in the form of testosterone oenanthate 250 mg intravenously each month. If this does not cause oedema or lead to an embarrassing or uncomfortable frequency of penile erection, the injections may be given every two weeks and continued at this rate, provided that they are well tolerated. The object of this treatment is to accelerate the rate of skeletal maturation so that the epiphyses fuse and further growth becomes impossible. Unfortunately, growth is accelerated in the early stages of treatment and the initial effect is therefore the opposite of that which the patient wishes. If he is already self-conscious about his stature, it may be more important to avoid further embarrassment at this stage than to reduce his height in adult life. This problem should be discussed carefully with the boy himself as well as his parents. He should also be warned of the slight risk that the treatment might impair fertility. The risk increases if the treatment is prolonged and it should not be continued for more than six months in the first instance. The whole problem should then be reassessed.

The treatment should begin before the secondary sex characters have developed beyond stage 3 of either genitalia or pubic hair. However, if it is begun at too early an age (i.e. before about 11 years) it may only add to the boy's psychological difficulties. The upper age limit for effective treatment with androgen is not known but it is unlikely that a useful result would be obtained if the skeletal age were greater than 14·0. It is impossible to predict how effective the treatment will be in an individual case.

Surgical. It is unlikely that this would be considered for a boy but the pros and cons would be the same as in the case of girls.

ERRATUM

Human Growth and its Disorders
W. A. Marshall

There is a potentially dangerous error on page 166, paragraph 4, line 2. The text reads "testosterone oenanthate 250 mg *intravenously* each month". This should read *intramuscularly* as intravenous injection of this substance could be highly dangerous.

References

Abrams, R. L., Grumbach, M. M. and Kaplan, S. L. (1971). *J. clin. Invest.* **50**, 940–950.

Baghdassarian, A., Guyda, H., Johanson, A., Migeon, C. J. and Blizzard, R. M. (1970). *J. clin. Endocr.* **31**, 428–435.

Bailey, J. A. (1973). "Disproportionate Short Stature; Diagnosis and Management." W. B. Saunders, Philadelphia.

Baker, G. L. (1969). *Amer. J. clin. Nutr.* **22**, 829–835.

Baker, P. T. (1969). *Science* **163**, 1149–1156.

Bayley, N. and Pinneau, S. R. (1952). *J. Pediat.* **40**, 423–441.

Björk, A. (1955). *Amer. J. Orthodont.* **41**, 198–225.

Brook, C. D. G., Lloyd, S. K. and Wolff, O. H. (1972). *Br. med. J.* **2**, 25–28.

Bruntland, G. H. and Walløe, L. (1973). *Nature*, **241**, 478–479.

Deming, J. (1957). *Hum. Biol.* **29**, 83–122.

Demirjian, A., Goldstein, H. and Tanner, J. M. (1973). *Hum. Biol.* **45**, 211–227.

Dewhurst, C. J. (1974). *Clinics. Obstet. Gynaec.* **1**, 619–647.

de Wijn, J. F. (1966). *in* "Somatic Growth of the Child" (J. J. van der Werff ten Bosch and A. Haak, eds.) pp. 16–23. Stenfert Kroese, Leiden.

Durnin, J. U. G. A. and Rahaman, M. M. (1967). *Br. J. Nutr.* **21**, 681–689.

Edwards, D. A. W., Hammond, W. H., Healy, M. J. R., Tanner, J. M. and Whitehouse, R. H. (1955). *Br. J. Nutr.* **9**, 133–143.

Faiman, C. and Winter, J. S. D. (1974). *in* "Control of the Onset of Puberty" (M. M. Grumbach, G. D. Grave and F. E. Mayer, eds.) pp. 32–61, Wiley, New York.

Filipsson, R. and Hall, K. (1975). *Ann. hum. Biol.* **2**, 355–363.

Finkelstein, J. W., Boyar, R. M., Roffwang, H., and Hellman, L. (1973). *Acta paediat. Scand.* **62**, 92.

Forsyth, C. C. (1974). *in* "Scientific Foundations of Paediatrics" (J. A. Davis and J. Dobbing, eds.) pp. 469–498, Heineman, London.

Friis-Hansen, B. J. (1957). *Acta paediat. Uppsala* Supplement 110.

Greulich, W. W. and Pyle, S. I. (1959). "Radiographic Atlas of Skeletal Development of the Hand and Wrist" Stanford University Press, California.

Grumbach, M. M., Roth, J. C., Kaplan, S. L. and Kelch, R. P. (1974). *in* "Control of the Onset of Puberty" (M. M. Grumbach, G. D. Grove, F. E. Mayer, eds. (pp. 115–166, Wiley, New York.

Gupta, D. (1975). *Clinics in Endocr. and Metab.* **4**, 27–56.

Gupta, D. and Marshall, W. A. (1971). *Acta Endocr.* **68**, 141–163.

Hall, K. (1971). *Acta Endocr.* **66**, 491–497.

Horton, R. and Tait, J. F. (1966). *J. clin. Invest.* **45**, 301–313.

Lee, M. C., Chang, K. S. F. and Chan, M. M. C. (1963). *Paediat.* **42**, 389–398.

Mahoudeau, J. A., Bardin, C. W. and Lipsett, M. B. (1971). *J. clin. Invest.* **50**, 1338–1344.

Maresh, M., and Groome, D. (1966). *Paediat.* **38**, 642–646.

Marshall, W. A. (1970). *in* "Brenneman's Practice of Paediatrics" (V. C. Kelley, ed.) Vol. 1, ch. 3, Harper and Row, University of Washington.

Marshall, W. A. (1974a). *Ann. hum. Biol.* **1**, 29–40.

Marshall, W. A. (1974b). *Clinics in Obstet. and Gynaec.* **1**, 593–618.

Marshall, W. A. (1975). *Ann. hum. Biol.* **2**, 243–250.

Marshall, W. A. and Limongi, Y. (1976). *Ann. hum. Biol.* **3**, 235–243.

Marshall, W. A. and Tanner, J. M. (1969). *Archs Dis. Childh.* **44**, 291–303.

Marshall, W. A. and Tanner, J. M. (1970). *Archs Dis. Childh.* **45**, 13–23.

Marshall, W. A., Ashcroft, M. T. and Bryan, G. (1970). *Hum. Biol.* **42**, 419–435.

Marubini, E. Resele, L. F., Tanner, J. M. and Whitehouse, R. H. (1972). *Hum. Biol.* **44**, 511–524.

McMahon, B. (1962). *J. nat. Cancer Inst.* **28**, 1173–1191.

Miller, R. W. (1956). *Paediatrics* **18**. 1–17.

Penrose, L. S. (1961). *in* "Recent Advances in Human Genetics" (L. S. Penrose, ed.) Little, Brown and Co., Boston.

Prokopec, M. (1965). *Acta Univ. Carol. Biol. Supplementum* 43–52.

Raiti, S., Johanson, A., Light, C., Migeon, C. J. and Blizzard, R. M. (1969). *Metabolism*, **18**, 234–240.

Rauh, J. and Schumsky, D. A. (1968). *in* "Human Growth" (D. B. Cheek, ed.) pp. 242–252, Lea and Febiger, Philadelphia.

Roberts, D. F. (1969). *J. biosoc. Sci. Supplement* **1**, 43–67.

Roberts, D. F. and Dann, T. C. (1967). *Br. J. prev. soc. Med.* **21**, 170–171.

Roche, A. F. and Wettenhall, H. N. B. (1969). *Aust. pediat. J.* **5**, 13–22.

Saez, J. M. and Morera, A. M. (1973). *Acta paediat. Scand.* **62**, 84.

Simmons, K. E. and Greulich, W. W. (1943). *J. Paediat.* **22**, 518–548.

Simon, G., Reid, L., Tanner, J. M., Goldstein, H., and Benjamin, B. (1972) *Archs Dis. Childh.* **47**, 373–381.

Singh, I. J., Savara, B. S. and Newman, M. T. (1967). *Hum. Biol.* **39**, 182–191.

Singleton, A., Patois, E., Pedion, G., and Roy, M. P. (1975). *Archs fr. Pédiat.* **32**, 859–869.

Siri, W. E. (1956). *in* "Advances in Biological and Medical Physics" (J. H. Lawrence and C. A. Tobias, eds.) Academic Press, New York.

Smith, D. W. (1970). "Recognisable Patterns of Human Malformation" B. W. Saunders, Philadelphia.

Sutow, W. W. and Conard, R. A. (1969). *in* "Radiation Biology of the Fetal and Juvenile mammal" (M. R. Sikov and D. D. Maklum, eds.) U.S. Atomic Energy Commission, Oak Ridge.

Tanner, J. M. (1962). "Growth at Adolescence" Blackwell Scientific Publications, Oxford.

Tanner, J. M. (1963). *Child Dev.* **34**, 817–848.

Tanner, J. M. (1965). *in* "Body Composition" Symposia of the Society for the Study of Human Biology, (G. A. Harrison, ed.) vol. 7, pp. 211–238, Pergamon Press, Oxford.

Tanner, J. M. (1972). *Nature* **237**, 431–437.

Tanner, J. M. (1973a). *in* "Textbook of Paediatrics" (J. O. Forfar and G. C. Arneil, eds) pp. 224–291, Churchill Livingstone, Edinburgh.

Tanner, J. M. (1973b). *Nature* **243**, 95–96.

Tanner, J. M. (1975). *in* "Endocrine and Genetic Diseases of Childhood and Adolescence" (L. I. Gardner, ed.) pp. 14–64, W. B. Saunders Co. Ltd.

Tanner, J. M. and Gupta, D. (1968). *J. Endocr.* **41**, 139–156.

Tanner, J. M. and Thomson, A. M. (1970). *Archs Dis. Childh.* **45**, 566–569.

Tanner, J. M. and Whitehouse, R. H. (1975). *Archs Dis. Childh.* **50**, 142–145.

Tanner, J. M. and Whitehouse, R. H. (1976). *Archs Dis. Childh.* **51**, 170–179.

Tanner, J. M., Whitehouse, R. H. and Takaishi, M. (1966). *Archs Dis. Childh.* **41**, 454–471; 613–635.

Tanner, J. M., Goldstein, H. and Whitehouse, R. H. (1970). *Archs Dis. Childh.* **45**, 755–762.

Tanner, J. M., Whitehouse, R. H., Hughes, P. C. R. and Vince, F. P. (1971). *Archs Dis. Childh.* **46**, 745–782.

Tanner, J. M., Lejarraga, H., and Cameron, N. (1975). *Paediat. Res.* **9**, 611–623.

Tanner, J. M., Whitehouse, R. H., Marshall, W. A., Healy, M. J. R. and Goldstein, H. (1975a). "Assessment of Skeletal Maturity and Prediction of Adult Height (TW2 method)" Academic Press, London.

Tanner, J. M., Whitehouse, R. H., Marshall, W. A. and Carter, B. S. (1975b). *Archs Dis. Childh.* **50**, 14–26.

Thomson, A. M. (1959). *Eugen. Rev.* **51**, 157–162.

Usher, R. H. and McLean, F. H. (1969). *J. Paediat.* **74**, 901–910.

van Wieringen, J. C., Wafelbakker, F., Vebrugge, H. P. and de Haas, J. H. (1968). "Groediagrammen Nederland, 1965" Wolters-Noordhoff n.v., Groningen.

Wettenhall, H. N. B., Cahill, C. and Roche, A. F. (1975). *Adol. Med.* **86**, 602–610.

Widdowson, E. M. (1951). *Lancet* **i**, 1316–1318.

Wilson, R. S. (1976). *Ann. hum. Biol.* **3**, 1–10.

Wilson, D. C. and Sutherland, I. (1949). *Br. med. J.* **2**, 130–132.

Yamazaki, J. M., Wright, S. W. and Wright, P. M. (1954). *J. Cell and Comp. Physiol.* **43**, suppl. I, 319–328.

Zachmann, M., Prader, A., Kind, H. R., Häfliger, H., and Budlinger, H. (1974). *Helv. paediat. Acta* **29**, 61–72.

Zachmann, M., Ferrandez, A., Mürset, G., and Prader, A. (1975). *Helv. paediat. Acta* **30**, 11–30.

Appendix

The following figures are enlarged versions of Figs. 20–23, reproduced here for practical use.

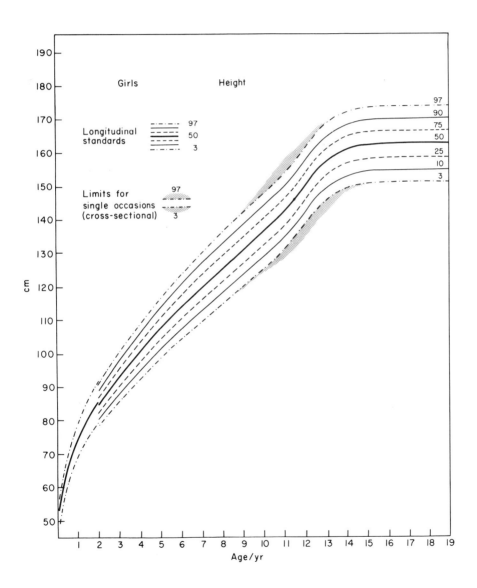

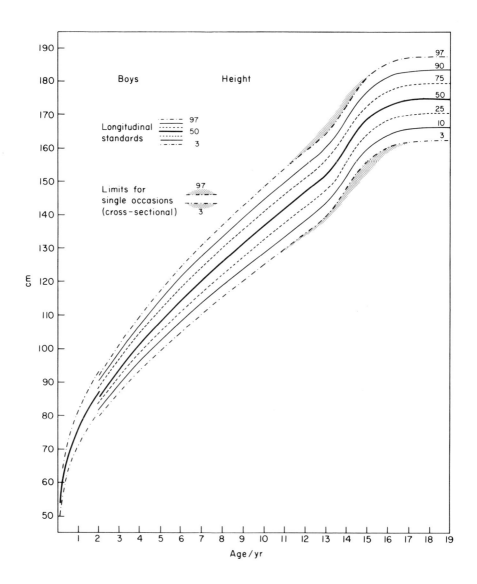

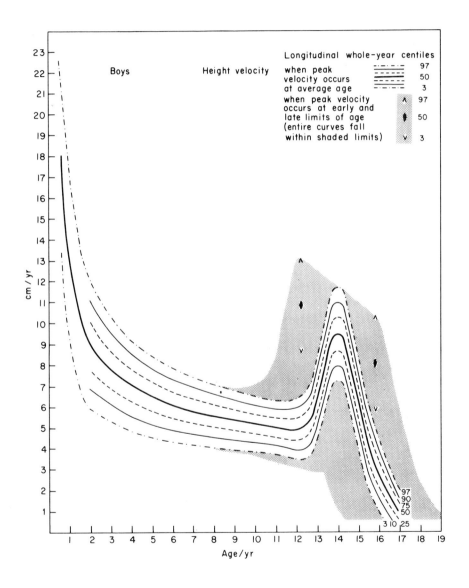

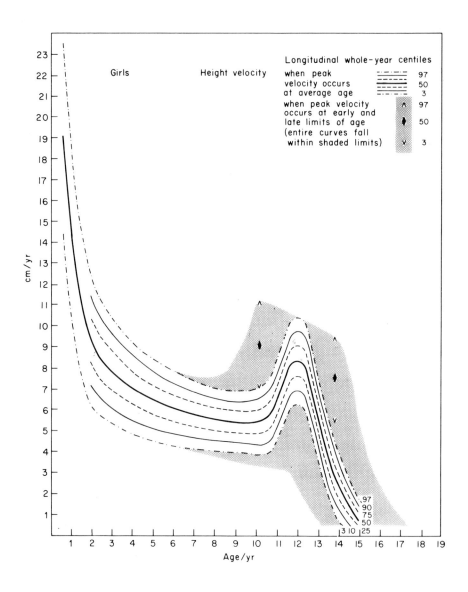

Subject Index